D1418303

DATE DUE

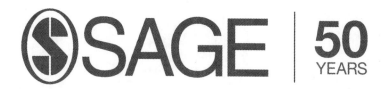

SAGE was founded in 1965 by Sara Miller McCune to support the dissemination of usable knowledge by publishing innovative and high-quality research and teaching content. Today, we publish more than 750 journals, including those of more than 300 learned societies, more than 800 new books per year, and a growing range of library products including archives, data, case studies, reports, conference highlights, and video. SAGE remains majority-owned by our founder, and after Sara's lifetime will become owned by a charitable trust that secures our continued independence.

Los Angeles | London | Washington DC | New Delhi | Singapore | Boston

Health Beliefs and Coping
with Chronic Diseases

Health Beliefs and Coping with Chronic Diseases

Ajit K Dalal

 SAGE www.sagepublications.com
Los Angeles • London • New Delhi • Singapore • Washington DC • Boston

First published in 2015 by

 SAGE Publications India Pvt Ltd
B1/I-1 Mohan Cooperative Industrial Area
Mathura Road, New Delhi 110 044, India
www.sagepub.in

SAGE Publications Inc
2455 Teller Road
Thousand Oaks, California 91320, USA

SAGE Publications Ltd
1 Oliver's Yard, 55 City Road
London EC1Y 1SP, United Kingdom

SAGE Publications Asia-Pacific Pte Ltd
3 Church Street
#10-04 Samsung Hub
Singapore 049483

Published by Vivek Mehra for SAGE Publications India Pvt Ltd, typeset in 10.5/12.5 pts Adove Garamond Pro by Diligent Typesetter, Delhi and printed at Chaman Enterprises, New Delhi.

Library of Congress Cataloging-in-Publication Data

Dalal, Ajit K., author.
    Health beliefs and coping with chronic diseases / Ajit K. Dalal.
       p.; cm.
    Includes bibliographical references and index.
    I. Title.
    [DNLM: 1. Chronic Disease—psychology. 2. Adaptation, Psychological. 3. Attitude to Health. 4. Complementary Therapies—psychology. 5. Culture. 6. Models, Psychological. WT 30]
    RC108   616'.044—dc23   2014044697

ISBN: 978-93-515-0078-0 (HB)

The SAGE Team: Shambhu Sahu, Alekha Chandra Jena, Rajib Chatterjee and Vinitha Nair

To
Jyoti, Shambhavi and Vibhu
who gave meaning to my life and work

Thank you for choosing a SAGE product! If you have any comment, observation or feedback, I would like to personally hear from you. Please write to me at <u>contactceo@sagepub.in</u>

—Vivek Mehra, Managing Director and CEO,
SAGE Publications India Pvt Ltd, New Delhi

Bulk Sales

SAGE India offers special discounts for purchase of books in bulk. We also make available special imprints and excerpts from our books on demand.

For orders and enquiries, write to us at

Marketing Department
SAGE Publications India Pvt Ltd
B1/I-1, Mohan Cooperative Industrial Area
Mathura Road, Post Bag 7
New Delhi 110044, India
E-mail us at <u>marketing@sagepub.in</u>

Get to know more about SAGE, be invited to SAGE events, get on our mailing list. Write today to <u>marketing@sagepub.in</u>

This book is also available as an e-book.

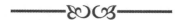

Contents

List of Tables   ix
Preface   xi
Acknowledgements   xiii

Unit I: Theory and Research
1. Psychology and Health: The Emerging Perspectives   3
2. Health Beliefs and Living with Chronic Diseases   25
3. Development of an Attribution Model of
   Psychological Recovery   50

Unit II: Beliefs about Chronic Diseases
4. Psychological Recovery of Accident Victims with
   Physical Disability   73
5. Health Beliefs and Psychological Adjustment to a
   Chronic Illness   86
6. Beliefs about the World and Recovery from
   Myocardial Infarction   99
7. Development of a Measure of Psychological Recovery   109
8. Measures of Perception of Hospital Environment and
   Affective Reactions   129

Unit III: Chronic Diseases, Self and Society
9. A Narrative Approach to Understand Illness Experience   153
10. Self-construal among Healthy and Chronically Sick Women   169

11. Family Support and Coping with Chronic Diseases   185
12. Folk Healing and Public Health-care Programmes   197

References   215
Index   238
About the Author   245

List of Tables

4.1 Psychological Stress Experienced by Patients with
   Temporary and Permanent Disability at Two Time Points   79
4.2 Frequency of Internal and External Causes   80
4.3 2 × 2 Analysis of Variance on the Cognitive Indices of
   Psychological Recovery   82
4.4 Correlations between Causal Attributions and
   Psychological Recovery   83
4.5 Correlation between Doctor's Assessment and
   Psychological Recovery   84

5.1 Correlations of Perceived Control and Psychological
   Adjustment with Causal and Recovery Beliefs   94

6.1 Partial Correlations of World, Causal and Recovery Beliefs
   for Physical and Psychological Recovery   105

7.1 Mean, SD, Cronbach Alphas (α) for All Four Subscales of
   Psychological Recovery and Their Correlations with
   Doctor's and Relative's Ratings   118
7.2 Intercorrelation among the Subscales of Psychological
   Recovery ($n = 80$)   119
7.3 Correlations of Background Characteristics with
   Measures of Psychological Recovery, Doctor's and
   Relative's Assessment   120
7.4 Mean Psychological Recovery of Four Categories of Patients   121

8.1 Perceived Hospital Environment Scale   139
8.2 Gender Differences in the Perception of
    Hospital Environment   140
8.3 Coping Responses to Hospitalization   141
8.4 Coping Responses across Nature of Health Problem
    and Gender   141
8.5 Correlations between Perceived Hospital Environment
    and Coping Responses   142

10.1 Demographic Background of Healthy and Chronically
    Sick Women   174

Preface

Study of cultural health beliefs has been an important stream of my research for the past quarter of a century. I have been engaged in examining how people suffering from chronic diseases perceive their disease, its causes and recovery. People do not view their health problem from medical perspective only but invoke a whole range of cultural beliefs to understand their predicament. How do these cultural beliefs about the disease and recovery shape a suffering person's affective reactions, expectations, initiatives and help-seeking behaviour? This volume is an anthology of studies in this area by the author and his colleagues.

Towards the end of 1984, I had to go through a major spinal surgery to deal with a life-threatening health condition. This gave me first-hand experience of how cultural beliefs contributed to my recovery from the surgery. As I was limping back to my academic job at the University, I was getting interested in research in this area. The first project I took up was on psychological recovery of the hospital patients suffering from some chronic condition. I conducted a series of studies on hospital patients, some of them with other colleagues, which were published in national and international journals. From these hospital studies, my interest grew in larger implications of cultural belief and in indigenous health practices in meeting health and well-being needs of people in a traditional society, like Indian. The endeavour was to show that people view health and illness from within a larger socio-cultural context, and understand the implications of their illness accordingly. These later studies are mostly of qualitative and conceptual nature.

In all, this volume comprises 12 chapters, divided into three units. These chapters, few of them reprinted from my published work, should provide insight into the salient role of cultural beliefs in understanding and managing health and well-being in the Indian context.

This volume should be an important reading for researchers in health and social sciences, who are interested in understanding health from a socio-cultural perspective. It should be of help in reformulating primary health care to render it compatible with cultural beliefs and practices.

Such a work cannot be completed without the support of many colleagues, friends and well-wishers. I acknowledge the help of all of them, without naming anyone in particular, who helped me in putting this volume together.

Ajit K Dalal

Acknowledgements

Permission from the publishers to reprint the following articles is acknowledged:

1. Dalal, A.K. and Singh, A.K. (1992). Role of causal and recovery beliefs in psychological adjustment to a chronic disease. *Psychology and Health: An International Journal*, 6, 193–203.
2. Agrawal, M. and Dalal, A.K. (1993). Beliefs about the world and recovery from myocardial infarction. *Journal of Social Psychology*, 133, 385–394.
3. Dalal, A.K. and Biswas, G. (2009). Self-construal among healthy and chronically sick women. *Psychological Studies*, 54(2), 142–149.
4. Dalal, A.K. (1995). Family support and coping with chronic diseases. *Indian Journal of Social Work*, 46, 167–176.
5. Dalal, A.K. and Pande, N. (1988). Psychological recovery of the accident victims with temporary and permanent disability. In Dalal, A.K. and Misra, G. (2002). *New Directions in Indian Psychology: Social Psychology*, vol. 1. New Delhi: SAGE Publications.

UNIT I

Theory and Research

1

Psychology and Health: The Emerging Perspectives

In the beginning of the last century, the field of health care grew around significant research in the area of bio-medicine. Development of antibiotics and other medicines led to the control of many epidemics, which were the major causes of human casualties and suffering. These new medicines also helped in dealing with a large number of infectious diseases and increasing longevity worldwide. Consequently, the physicians and medical hospitals come to dominate the field of health. Medical practitioners were at the helm of decision-making about people's health and controlled health-care systems all over the world. It was in the last quarter of the past century that a realization started building up that health is a much broader concept than was conceived by the modern medicine. It was dawning on researchers that health and illness cannot be viewed merely as bodily states but also implicate psychological, social and cultural aspects of human existence. An eminent Chilean philosopher and activist Ivan Ellich (1974) concluded that health is too important to be left in the charge of medical practitioners only. It encompasses the family and social life of a person and is, therefore, a collective responsibility of all social institutions.

Recent research and writings based on cumulative evidences have led to two general conclusions. First, cultural beliefs shape health behaviour. People construct their understanding of the world, including their beliefs about medicine and disease from their interaction with cultural institutions, social groups and divinity. Consequently, the way people understand their own and other's illness, take remedial measures, comply with treatment regimen and cope with health crises are largely shaped by the culture they belong to. Evidently, medicine, health care, illness and doctor–patient relationship are cultural activities and experiences, and, as such, are legitimate areas of study for social scientists. The socio-cultural aspects of medicine and health-related knowledge and practices as interpreted within the epistemological traditions of a society provide the basis for patients' responses to various diseases. Healing institutions and health care in any society are, in effect, natural products of prevalent cultural beliefs and practices (Lupton, 1994). Social scientists are still grappling to fully comprehend the socio-cultural aspects of medicine.

The second conclusion, already known in all traditional societies but rediscovered in the medical field, is that there is a close symbiotic relationship between the mind and the body. Even though a disease may be a bodily affliction, mental states are important factors in causing, as well as in recovering from the disease. The rapid growth of modern medicine has primarily relied on the Descartian logic of mind–body dualism and on a mechanistic view of the human life. As a consequence, modern medicine primarily deals with removal of the disease as pathology of the human body. There are mounting empirical evidences that mind and body are intimately linked with each other and that one cannot be treated without treating the other. This acknowledgement of close interaction between the mental and the physical worlds has further expanded the domain of health by encompassing thoughts, feelings, lifestyle and social relations. In essence, health has come to imply not only the physical but also social, psychological and spiritual well-being.

It is no surprise that the Descartian psychology did not show much interest in physical health, which was considered a field of medical sciences. Psychological researches were primarily concerned with mental health problems. Consequently, clinical psychologists restricted themselves to investigate the aetiology of mental illnesses, and to diagnose and treat such patients. Emphasis has been on examining stressful life experiences and their psychological consequences. Clinical psychologists confined psychotherapeutic treatment to patients with varied mental health problems. Even here, their role remained subsidiary to psychiatrists. This clear demarcation between mental and physical health was consistent with the notion of mind–body dualism. Thus, from the beginning clinical psychology did not deal with somatic problems. The concepts, theories and methods of clinical psychology were ill-equipped to handle somatic health problems. A new psychology was to begin to treat and augment somatic health. This is how health psychology began to grow as a field distinct from clinical psychology. The emerging discipline of health psychology got recognition only in 1970s and the first journal in the area of *Health Psychology* was started in 1982. In present times, health psychology is one of the most rapidly growing disciplines in psychology.

In the last two decades, psychological factors have come to be identified as major causes of a wide range of physical diseases and disabilities. For example, Type A personality (impatient, ambitious, impersonal, etc.) is considered a major risk factor in heart diseases. Prolonged psychological stress is found to be responsible for hypertension, peptic ulcer and many other diseases. Again, psychological factors have also been found important in recovering from these physical diseases. In recent times, the role of health psychologists is increasingly acknowledged in the treatment of somatic diseases. Patient compliance, doctor–patient communication, attitude change and self-care are some of the areas in which health psychologists can make important contributions. Furthermore, cultural factors such as social beliefs, values and practices need to be examined, both in maintaining good health and causing illnesses (Dalal, 2005; Joshi, 2000; Sharma and Misra, 2012). The scope of health psychology is now expanding in promoting health and in making preventive health measures effective. Psychological rehabilitation of patients with chronic diseases and disabilities is another field that is gaining popularity.

In the backdrop of such evidences of psychological factors playing an important role in enhancing physical health, the biomedical model of health care is under serious scrutiny. It seems to be of limited use in dealing with the expanding domain of health and cannot by itself succeed in bringing a sick person back to normal life routine. The alternative psychomedical model, as enunciated in this volume, is claimed to have greater viability in improving the health status of people in any society. In this introductory chapter, we will first examine biomedical model, explore the psychological factors associated with health and illness, and then examine the efficacy of the proposed psychomedical model of patient care.

The Biomedical Model of Health Care

The biomedical model has governed the thinking of most health practitioners for the last one and half centuries in the west. It has now got worldwide acceptance and has been adopted as an official health-care programme by almost all countries. India is no exception where health policies and programmes have primarily relied on biomedical model. The vast network of hospitals, dispensaries and down to primary health centres are manned by professionals trained in the biomedical tradition.

The biomedical model considers disease as a biological malfunctioning—some kind of biochemical imbalance or neurophysiological disturbance. In this, the body is held as a machine that can be analysed in terms of parts, that is, a system of synchronized organs. A disease is seen as impaired functioning of a biological mechanism and the doctor's role is to intervene, either physically or chemically, to rectify malfunctioning of the specific body parts (Capra, 1982). The model is based on the assumption of mind–body dualism in which psychological and social processes are considered independent of the disease process. Though the emotional state of the patient is considered important, it is kept outside the purview of medical treatment (Taylor, 2006).

Historically, the biomedical model is a logical outgrowth of the philosophical and scientific developments in Europe in the age of enlightenment. It is consistent with the individualistic and capitalistic worldview of the post-industrial societies. The biomedical theory of disease grew around the conviction that most diseases are caused by invaders from the outside 'microorganisms or germs'. The discovery of antibiotics in the 1930s and 1940s gave impetus to modern medicine; the 'miracle drugs' seized public imagination. There were great hopes that medical science would eventually discover an effective drug therapy to eradicate every known disease; that, there will be 'a pill for every ill'. This belief was so strong that even emotional and mental disorders were treated with various drugs, ignoring their psychogenic antecedents. The biomedical model of health care has not fulfilled the expectations it aroused. Adherence to this model has helped in reducing mortality by controlling prevalence of contagious diseases. The life span at birth is increasing all over the world (between 60 and 80 years in different countries), though the actual contribution of biomedicine towards this success is debated.

Improved economic status, social hygiene and health consciousness have also made significant difference.

Apart from the growing disillusionment, the biomedical model has serious limitations in terms of health practices. The model treats a patient as an organism, a biological phenomenon. The proponents of this model were more interested in the disease than the patient. Thus, when the curative aspect is taken up, the emphasis is on the nature of diseases, its various symptoms and on the ways to remove them. In this process, the patient is only a recipient of certain medication, taking no cognizance of the psychological state of the patient. Biomedical practices envisage no role for the patient and his or her support group in diagnosis and in deciding about the course of treatment. The interest in the patient as a person is just incidental. As Siegel (1986) observed '... (medical) practitioners still act as though disease catches people, rather than understanding that people catch disease by becoming susceptible to the germs of the illness to which we are constantly exposed' (p. 2). Thus, most of the health schemes focus on providing better medical facilities rather than involving the patient towards a common goal of attending sickness. Quite often medical practitioners learn from their personal experiences that diagnosis would be more accurate and treatment more effective if the patient's socio-economic background, beliefs, needs and anxieties are also taken into consideration. Nevertheless, it is presumed that the patient would be receptive, willing to supply all necessary information and would conform to the treatment regimen. This may be so, at the most, in case of hospitalized patients. In cases of chronic diseases particularly, patients and their families do not always accept the passive role and frequently engage in their own, at times, 'in some secret forms of curing', depending on their appraisal of the disease and its future course (Engel, 1977). The biomedical model views with scepticism the practices of faith and spiritual healing, and with that all the cultural traditions of managing health problems.

The biomedical model breaks down when it comes to preventive health care, where there are no cooperative-captive patients; where people are under no compulsion to comply with health procedures. People may even pay no heed when they are told about the adverse health consequences of some of their habits, like smoking. There may be differences in the phenomenological meanings of illness and health. In brief, unless people are willing to cooperate, no preventive health care is possible.

Psychosomatic Illness

The existing medical practices have, in reality, not completely ignored the psychological basis of many diseases such as ulcers, coronary heart diseases, bronchitis and hypertension. The causal connection between mental disorders and physical diseases is a subject of serious discussion within biomedical sciences. The diseases that have psychogenic base are called psychosomatic diseases. This branch of medicine, though acknowledges that many diseases are caused by psychological factors, yet makes no distinction in terms of treatment.

Psychological stress is considered to be the main cause of psychosomatic diseases. What does a stressful life event do to a person? Selye (1976) has argued for a three-phase reaction to psychological stress. First is the alarm phase, during which people mobilize all their social and psychological resources to combat the threat. In the second phase, people make efforts to cope with the threat, as through confrontation. In the third phase, exhaustion occurs if people fail to overcome the threat and deplete their physical resources. This could lead to the onset of physical symptoms. Much depends on how an individual appraises the stressors, and on the social support and intrapersonal resources available to a person (Lazarus, 1966; Mason, 1971). In the latter work, Lazarus (2000) showed much interest in cataclysmic events that have sudden and powerful impact on health status. Events like natural disasters (flood, cyclone), accidents and life-threatening diseases (heart disease, cancer, AIDS) are unpredictable but may result in serious crisis for the person. People show all kinds of physical symptoms while going through such life crises. Coping in such cases is long term and there may be no immediate recovery.

Presently, psychological stress is a fast-growing area of research and there is a tendency to view many illnesses as psychosomatic. Though there is some understanding of the psychological factors causing physiological problems, there is little success in finding effective treatment for many psychosomatic diseases. The result is that most physicians continue to fall back on their biomedical model to evolve a course of treatment by prescribing drugs. In brief, psychological data are used to understand the aetiology of diseases but this has no bearing on the course of treatment, which is primarily drug therapy.

The Second World War was an immense human tragedy, and provided overbearing evidences of the effects of psychological traumas on physical health. In a large number of hospitals, separate departments of 'psychosomatic medicine' were started. These departments aimed to understand, for example, how episodes of anger and hostility can translate into stomach ulcers and heart attacks. But, because medicine so rigidly compartmentalized the realms of mind and body this new discipline never got the respect it deserved (Benson, 1997). In the long run, this may have been for the best as obviously no one discipline can address the complex inter-relatedness of the mind and the body. Subsequently, in clinical practices, both in medical and clinical psychology, the classification of diseases as 'psychosomatic' was seriously questioned; so much so that in later versions of DSM the category of 'psychosomatic' diseases is eliminated. Instead, the term 'somatoform illnesses' is more popular as an international diagnostic category (ICD).

In 1955, Beecher, a surgeon, wrote a paper in the Journal of the American Medical Association titled 'The Powerful Placebo'. In this paper he concluded, that '35% of a drug's or a doctor's success is due to patient's expectation of a desired outcome, or the placebo response' (Beecher, 1955, p. 1602). He inferred this on the basis of his experience during the Second World War and a review of 15 published intervention studies. Despite later criticism about soundness of the applied methodology, this paper is still one of the most cited publications on placebo effect. It is a well-known fact that physicians very often use placebo drugs to treat their patients when they think that patients' symptoms have no organic base, or when doctors are not sure what treatment will work and want to give an impression to the patients that drugs are prescribed to control their problem. Such placebos could be vitamin or other tablets without any active chemical agent. Surprisingly, quite often the results of placebo drugs are as good as that of actual drugs, much to the embarrassment of the attending physician. There is resistance to acknowledge that body's own healing system works, and that a positive mental state can cure a psychosomatic illness.

Research on placebo's effect has primarily focused on expectations as the key factor. In general, expectation is aimed at preparing the body to anticipate an event in order to better cope with it. For example, the expectation of a negative outcome results in anticipating a possible threat, thus increasing anxiety, whereas the expectation of a positive outcome may reduce anxiety and activate the corresponding neuronal networks (Benedetti, 2011; Price et al., 2008).

Acknowledging that placebo works is akin to accepting that psychological interventions are effective. Though our knowledge of when and how placebos work across different disease conditions and therapeutic interventions is still very limited. We need to identify different social, psychological and neurobiological determinants of placebo effects in different chronic diseases, at different stages. It is also important to know why placebos work in case of some patients and not in the other. Without proper understanding of the diseased people and their sociopsychological context administration of placebo may be hazardous also. However, studies of placebo effects provide important understanding of the role of beliefs in dealing with physical diseases.

Stress and Body's Immune System

There is increasing evidence that grief, depression and other negative feelings are linked with the increased risk of organic (like cancer) and infectious (like cold) diseases. For example, recent bereavement has been linked with the increased risk of a number of diseases, such as coronary heart disease, tuberculosis, allergies and peptic ulcers (Clegg, 1988; Cohen and Herbert, 1996). In recent years, a new field of pyschoneuroimmunology has emerged to examine the mediating role of psychological factors in immune deficiency. The body's immune system is presumed to be interacting with the central nervous system and endocrine system on one hand, and with psychological and social factors on the other hand. It is important to bear in mind that significant individual differences exist in the manner and extent to which stress is perceived, processed and coped with. Stress-related negative emotions tend to suppress body's immune system over an extended time, rendering the person vulnerable to a host of diseases.

The immune system protects the body from the invading microorganisms—bacteria, virus, fungi and parasites. These are called antigens. The immune system of the body, rather than being a centralized system, operates through a blood circulatory process throughout the body and gets activated wherever antigens are encountered. Called lymphocytes, these are special types of white blood cells, medically termed

T cells, B cells and NK (natural killer) cells. These blood cells multiply, differentiate and mature in bone marrows, thymus, lymph nodes, spleen and other body parts. The lymphocytes produce their own antigens to mobilize a direct attack to kill the invading foreign microorganisms in the blood stream. Glasser (1996) pointed out that the immune system must be extraordinarily efficient in destroying the invading bacteria and viruses on an ongoing basis to keep us healthy. Beginning soon after birth, there is a steady decrease in the ability of thymus gland to produce new ('naïve') white blood cells (T lymphocytes, or 'T cells'), with a substantial reduction by age 50 and almost complete incapacity by age 60 (Parham, 2005). One result is that older individuals have a greater percentage of memory T cells, which have been trained to respond to a particular pathogen (adaptive immune system), than the naïve T cells, which can respond to a novel invader. Still adaptive immune system takes several days to engage but is more efficient and effective once activated (Gomez et al., 2005). It is only when the body's immune system is destroyed by a virus called human immunodeficiency virus (HIV) that people become highly vulnerable to all kinds of infections.

At times, acute stress can augment lymphocyte maturation or function in ways that can enhance innate and adaptive immunity. This suggests that depending on the condition under which the immune response is initiated, stress can enhance the acquisition and expression of immunoprotection and immunopathology. In contrast to acute stress, chronic stress suppresses or dysregulates innate and adaptive immune responses. More chronic the stress is, more severe is the damage caused to the immune system. Kiecolt-Glaser and Glaser (2002) reported that examination stress results in poorer immunocompetence, more so for lonely students. Kiecolt-Glaser et al. (1987) found that women who were recently separated had lower immunity than married women. Willis et al. (1987) conducted a longitudinal study in which 15 healthy elderly people facing major life crisis (like accident, bereavement, etc.) were given many physiological measures over a long period. The analysis of the data revealed that in their case lymphatic concentration, caloric intake and body weight decreased, whereas cortisol concentration increased soon after the crisis. More recently, in a meta-analytic study of more than 300 empirical articles describing a relationship between psychological stress and parameters of the immune system in human participants was conducted by Segerstrom and Miller (2004). It was found that acute stressors (lasting for a very short time) were associated with potentially adaptive up-regulation of some parameters of natural immunity and down-regulation of some functions of specific immunity. Brief naturalistic stressors (such as exams) tended to suppress cellular immunity while preserving humoral immunity. It is chronic, enduring stress, which is associated with suppression of both cellular and humoral measures, and thus particularly problematic (Cohen, 2005).

The effect of stress on the body's immune functioning is, however, mediated by a number of factors, including nature and severity of stressors. For example, the stressors that are uncontrollable produce more adverse effects than those that are controllable. Again, people who were more depressed were found to be more susceptible to infectious diseases and showed slower recovery rate. Schleifer et al. (1989, 1993) discovered on the basis of empirical work and meta-analysis that depression was associated with immunodepression, primarily among older and hospitalized patients. Also, a mild physical stress experienced in the recent past may enhance immunity against the adverse effects of the present stress experience.

However, not much is still known about the possible physical mechanism through which psychosocial factors play the influencing role. Several lines of work suggest that psychosocial stress alters the composition of brain chemicals, triggering chain reactions in the central nervous system and the hypothalamus, which regulates the secretions of the endocrine system and increases the level of corticoid in the blood. The corticoid in the blood is presumed to damage lymphocytes and lower the efficiency of the immune system. Chronic stresses, negative emotions and lack of social support often silently block the breeding of NK cells in the blood. These findings are, however, suggestive of the possible linkages and could be mediated by a large number of concomitant factors (Segerstrom and Miller, 2004).

Psychological Antecedents of Physical Diseases

Apart from lowering body's immune functioning, psychosocial factors directly influence physical health. A broad range of social, cultural and psychological variables have been linked with the onset and course of many chronic diseases. Health practitioners have been aware of these factors since time immemorial, and were accounting for these factors in their curative, preventive and promotive health prescriptions. Research evidences accumulated in last 2–3 decades substantiate that psychological stress and dispositional factors cause chronic diseases, such as hypertension, cancer, heart disease and ulcers.

A number of socio-psychological factors having implications for health include health-impairing habits (smoking, alcoholism), family and work environment, dietary habits, and lifestyle. Cultural factors play an important role in shaping many health-related behaviours, which are discussed in more detail in Chapter 2. Here, we will primarily confine to person-related factors and their linkages with health and illness.

Stressful Life Events

Be it a failure in an examination or an interview, or the death of someone near and dear, all of us have experienced such tragic events in our lives and usually cope with them successfully. Of course, this is not true with everyone, every time. It is now well established that the mortality rate is much higher among widows and widowers than among married persons of the same age. Young et al. (1963), for example, found a sharp rise in mortality rate during the first 6 months of widowerhood. Talbott et al. (1981) examined the medical records of 80 women who died suddenly of heart attack. In comparison to a control group of sample, these women had twice more often experienced the death of a close relative or friend within six months of their fatal heart attack.

The pioneering work of Selye (1976) has suggested that stressful events lead to health-impairing physiological changes and illness. People fall ill because of some kind of pressure their lives go through. Following Selye's work, stress was defined in medical science as a specific physiological condition, the *general adaptation syndrome*. This syndrome or physiological change is caused by the person's own adaptive response to the stresses experienced. This means that although the syndrome itself is specific (specific changes in bodily systems), the condition of stress it results in is a generalized state of the person (Radleys, 1994).

Hinkle (1973) further extended Selye's biological model of stress by adding two more points. The first is that stress works through the central nervous system. This means that the relationship of a stressor to the internal state is contingent on the meaning of that event for the person. The second point is that stress engenders changes to which a person must adapt. It was suggested that change is an essential aspect of life, so that it is hard to conceive of a state of stress which is qualitatively different from any other state of being alive. The experienced stress thus affects general health status by lowering immunity, rather than causing a specific disease. Despite intense research activity in this area a clear relationship between stress and disease is yet to be established. Many factors mediate responses to stressful conditions.

Though Selye did not test his model empirically, his work aroused much interest in this field. Holmes and Rahe (1967) developed a measure of overall stress due to life events. They tried to establish linkages between the level of stress and strain (physical, psychosomatic and mental health). The Schedule of Recent Experiences developed by them is a self-administered questionnaire containing 43 life events to which subjects responded by checking those events that they have experienced in the recent past (six months to one year). The schedule was based on the rational that life changes per say are stressful, regardless of the desirability of the event experienced. More than 300 such scales were developed since the publication of Holmes and Rahe's scale but no clear-cut pattern of any relationship between life events and strain has emerged. Many scales developed later separately examined positive and negative events. A measure of negative events was found to be a better predictor of strain than just a change measure (Agrawal and Naidu, 1988). As Lindsey (1993) correctly noted, however, it is not possible to capture the proposed *stress response* and its magnitude by such measures alone.

One of the reasons for the lack of a linear relationship between life stressors and illness could be the respondents' own appraisal orientation. Lazarus (1966, 1984) posits that a stressful life event can be appraised as potentially harmful (as with illness and injury), or threatening (to self-esteem), or challenging (offering opportunity for gain and growth). Such differential appraisal of the same stressor gives rise to different emotions and coping responses. When the appraisal of threat persists in the face of failure to cope with the stress, it leads to greater incidents of diseases.

Because of this failure to establish a clear relationship between stressful life events and illness, many researchers have shifted their attention to the study of daily hassles, which seems to have a cumulative effect on the occurrence of chronic diseases. Major life events occur less frequently and tend to have a more distal impact on well-being and physical health, whereas daily stressors tend to have a more proximal effect (Almeida, 2005). Furthermore, the two types of stressors may interact, such that the impact of daily stressors may be magnified in the context of exposure to negative life events. Daily hassles are stable, repetitive, low intensity problems encountered in daily life. The impact of these low intensity stresses persists. Their effect on body systems is gradual but in long term, may be more damaging than the cataclysmic events. Noise, environmental pollution, job dissatisfaction and crowded neighbourhood are few examples of such daily hassles. In a study of Navajo Indians in New Mexico, USA (Williams et al., 1992), it was observed that people scoring high on life events and daily hassles were more prone to falling ill in the near future. Records of the only hospital in that area were checked two years after the administration of these scales. It was discovered that a relative excess of daily irritants (hassles) over pleasant experiences was associated with an increased risk of hospitalization. High level of daily hassles was found to be a significant predictor of increased utilization of out-patient services.

Cognitive Orientation

As stated by Lazarus (1984), people construe a stressful life event in their own idiosyncratic ways. Many studies have focused on the manner in which people appraise the severity of the events, its causal explanations and ramifications. Some people are more negative in their subjective construction of the event, view the situation as uncontrollable and feel helpless and hopeless. Abramson et al. (1978) postulated a pessimistic explanatory style, characterized by internal (self), stable and global explanations of the negative events. In a meta-analysis of 104 studies on about 15,000 subjects, Sweeney et al. (1986) found a highly stable relationship between pessimistic explanatory style and depression. In a 35-year longitudinal study, Peterson et al. (1988) found that pessimistic explanatory style was not linked with poor health at the age of 25, but significantly predicted poor health above the age of 45 years. One explanation given was that at a young age people have physical resources to absorb negativity, but these get depleted as age advances.

Positive orientation or thinking about the crisis is another important cognition that has wide implications for recovery from any disease. Studies (Scheier and Carver, 1985; Scheier et al., 1986) have shown that optimism (generalized expectancy of good outcomes) is associated with problem-focused coping, seeking social support, seeing the positive side of the illness and accepting uncontrollable outcomes. Optimistic beliefs are specifically beneficial when patients suffer from a chronic disease that is to a considerable extent controllable (Fournier, de Ridder and Bensing, 2002; Giltay et al., 2006). Taylor (1983) observed that positive comparison was often used by cancer patients for self-enhancement in the event of an accident or illness. The patients who compared themselves with those who were in worse conditions recovered earlier. In a study by Agrawal et al. (1994), positive life orientation was found to be an important predictor of medical, as well as, of psychological recovery of myocardial patients. Positive life orientation also predicts good survival prognosis in old age (Tilvis et al., 2012).

Personality Dispositions

Personality dispositions were also found to have significant bearings on health status. Many personality traits predispose an individual to a negative emotional state, such as depression, anxiety and nervousness, or lead to maladaptive coping behaviours. Mathews and Ridgeway (1981) identified a large number of personality variables associated with surgical recovery. Feeling of control and positive attitude were found to be important factors in the success of surgery (Hunt et al., 1984). Also, recovery of the surgical patients was found to be contingent on patient's emotional state prior to the surgery (see Cohen and Lazarus, 1979).

One such personality variable is Type A behaviour pattern that significantly contributes to the occurrence of coronary heart disease (Jenkins, 1974; Glass, 1976). A Type A person shows extreme competitiveness, a sense of urgency (always feels rushed or is impatient when delayed), excessive involvement in work, aggressiveness and hostility. Individuals displaying this behaviour pattern seem to be engaged in chronic, ceaseless and unnecessary struggle with themselves, with others and with circumstances. In contrast, Type B behaviour pattern is characterized by a low level of competitiveness, time urgency and hostility. They are easygoing and philosophical. In a study of eight-and-half-year follow-up of more than 5,000 people, Rosenman et al. (1970) confirmed that Type A behaviour is strongly related to coronary heart disease incidence. The mortality from this disease was twice as high in Type A patients than in Type B patients. Their study revealed that those who exhibited competitive lifestyles were more likely to develop coronary heart disease (myocardial infarction, angina pretoris and silent heart attack) even when biological risk factors (like smoking) were controlled. Weiss and Lonnquist (1996) suggested three possible mediators between Type A behaviour and heart disease—(a) some underlying physical weakness may be associated with Type A behaviour, (b) hyper-responsivity of Type A person may cause over-activity of sympathetic nervous system and (c) Type A behaviour leads to more risky circumstances, such as delay in treatment. However, some studies (Gallacher et al., 2003) found both confirmatory and null results taking Type A behaviour pattern. Bhattacharyya (2001), taking a sample from Kolkata, found clear evidence that chronic heart disease patients were competitive, hyper-alert and tense.

A similar search for a cancer-prone personality has also not been very successful. There is some evidence that those who develop cancer are unable to express positive feelings (Soloman, 1969), make an extensive use of repressive and make less use of ego defence. Longer survival rate among cancer patients was associated with more frequent expression of hostility and other negative feelings (Derogatis, 1991). A new personality pattern known as Type C (cancer-prone) has been identified by psychologists, which responds to stress with depression and a sense of hopelessness. Type C personalities have a tendency to be introverted, respectful, eager to please, conforming and compliant. Type C people are basically nice guys who never show anger and other negative reactions in public. They are helping, cooperative, smiling type, never hurting others but at the same time never expressing their true feelings. These are lonely people, even shy of seeking help when need be. Derogatis discovered that Type C people have four times higher risk of cancer than others.

Still another personality pattern, termed as Type D personality was reported to be closely linked with high rate of mortality by Denollet (2000). According to Denollet (2000, 2004), Type D personality comprises two broad and stable traits—(a) negative affectivity—people who have greater tendency to experience negative feelings. People high on this trait often feel unhappy, tend to worry, are depressed, easily irritable, and lack self-esteem and assertiveness. (b) Social inhibition-tendency to inhibit feelings and behaviour in social situation. Such people are reserved, lack social support and avoid intimacy (Pederson et al., 2006). Denollet (2004) predicted that such personality may aggravate disease directly through pathophysiological mechanism. It is quite likely that Type D personality may precipitate heart attack as well as many other fatal diseases. A close link of Type D personality with peripheral arterial diseases (Emons et al., 2012) and health status of patients with cardiac defibrillators (Pedersen et al., 2012) has been established.

Along similar lines, Suzanne Kobasa (1979) proposed a positive personality type called *hardiness*, to differentiate people who do and who do not get sick under prolonged stress. Hardiness includes three characteristics: (1) personal control—people's belief that they can influence events in their lives, (2) commitment—people's sense or purpose of involvement in events, activities and people in their lives, and (3) challenge—tendency to view changes as opportunities to growth rather than as threat to security. Hardy people are better able to deal with stressors and are less likely to fall sick. Kobasa (1979) in a study of highly stressful executives found that those who fall sick were those who scored low on hardiness scale. However, because of the correlational nature of most of these studies it is not yet ruled out that it is illness, which could be shaping hardiness.

A construct closely related to hardiness but different enough to be a powerful mediator between life events of stress and illness is *sense of coherence* (SOC) (Antonovsky, 1988). SOC is characterized by (a) comprehensibility—the degree to which a situation is predictable and explicable, (b) manageability—the availability of sufficient resources (internal and external) to meet the demands of the situation and (c) meaningfulness—the degree to which life's demands are worthy of the investment of energy. Persons with a high SOC have a tendency to view the world as ordered, predictable and manageable. Importantly, Antonovsky (1988) argued that we often ask the wrong question—that is, 'Why do some people become ill?'—when, perhaps we should be asking, 'Why do people stay healthy despite life stresses?'

Psychomedical Approach to Patient Care

The research discussed above make it abundantly clear that psychosocial factors are important considerations in all health-care programmes. Physical ailment is only one aspect of the illness experience, which is also psychosocial in nature. With the failure of the biomedical system in meeting health needs and alleviating human suffering, the search for some alternative models is still on. To account for the interplay of biological, psychological and social factors in the domain of health, many health psychologists have proposed the biopsychosocial model as an alternative to biomedical model (Engel, 1977; Shorter, 2005). The biopsychosocial model emphasizes the symbiotic relation between mind and body in influencing the health status of an individual. To integrate micro-level processes of biological factors with the macro-level psychosocial factors, this model takes a system approach to health and illness. The system approach maintains that biological and psychosocial factors are hierarchically organized. Consequently, preventive–promotive health and illness are considered interrelated and integrated domains within the individuals. However, in this biopsychosocial model there is preponderance of biomedical practices and psychosocial components are considered subservient to them. In this, health and clinical psychologists are only supportive members of the team of medical practitioners to prevent diseases and in planning the course of treatment. Contemporary psychiatry has primarily developed on the ideology of biopsychosocial model. This model was popularized in the USA and coincided with the publication of DSM-III and beginning of psychopharmacology. It helped in maintaining the hegemony of medical professionals. Public health issues are thus largely managed by medical professionals, so much so that the WHO is primarily dominated by medical experts. The biopsychosocial model, which was promoted in reaction to medical reductionism, has played out its role and the search is still on to find more viable approaches to health and illness (Ghaeml, 2009).

Building on an alternative approach, a new model of health care is proposed in this and subsequent chapters. Referred to as the *psychomedical model of health care*, it emphasizes on the greater salience on psychological aspects of the illness than on medical aspects. In a broader sense, psychological factors are considered to influence promotional, preventive and curative aspects of the health. In this, the distinction between mental and physical health is considered to be a matter of practical consideration only. In the specific context of physical illness, this approach acknowledges that emotional and mental interventions can bring a person back to normal health in most of the cases, with or without medical intervention. There are recursive causal linkages between psychological and biological states of a person. Consequently, the recovery process is considered incomplete until one has recovered both psychologically and physically.

Health is a multidimensional phenomenon, in which a balance of physical, social and psychological aspects of one's existence is an important consideration. It is quite likely that physical disease may be balanced by a positive mental attitude and social support, so that the overall state is that of well-being. On the other hand, emotional problems or social isolation can make a person sick in spite of physical fitness. Of course, this balance is dynamic and not a static equilibrium. It acknowledges an individual's ability to adapt to environmental changes and an innate tendency to re-establish oneself in a balanced state when it is disturbed. From the psychomedical point of view, health is seen as an experience of well-being resulting from a dynamic balance that involves the physical and psychological aspects of the organism, as well as its interaction with its natural and social environment.

The basic assumption of the psychomedical approach is the *unity* of the mind and body. As far as the state of health is concerned, it is not possible to distinguish and separate the contribution of mind and body. This inseparable nature of mind–body was well accepted in all ancient societies of east and west. Patients were treated not only by the physicians but by healers, religious people and by others. It was only towards the 17–18th century that in the West with the emphasis on scientific approach, mind, which was thought to be associated with consciousness and soul, was rejected as a legitimate domain of study in modern medicine. The Cartesian principle accepted the mind–body dualism that mental processes do not affect somatic processes. Scientific evidences have now accumulated that not only mind and body are closely interlinked, but that mind has a capacity to heal the body.

The psychomedical model views the patient as a person embedded in a socio-cultural context, in which he or she imbibes certain belief system. These socio-cultural beliefs would determine the way a patient evaluates and attributes meaning to one's sickness. Kleinman (1986) has made a distinction in his research between disease and illness. Whereas disease is an organic malfunctioning as diagnosed by a medical practitioner, illness is a subjective construction of the experience of a disease by the patient. It is patient's own interpretation and perception of the disease, which is greatly influenced by the culture to which the patient belongs. In a traditional society like India, an illness is a social event, which not only concerns the patient, but also his or her family, friends, relations and others in the social network. Everyone joins in appraising the illness (Dalal and Misra, 2006).

Patients' phenomenology, that is, their attitudes, values and beliefs are crucial in deciding about the type of treatment sought and the extent to which people would comply the curative regime. According to the Health Belief Model propounded by Rosenstock (1966, 1974), knowledge of patient's health-related beliefs is crucial in understanding the patient's psychological state of readiness to take specific action. For example, patients' compliance can be predicted considering their beliefs about severity, susceptibility and consequences of an illness, as well as cost of a regimen and its likelihood of success (Becker and Maiman, 1975). Rosenstock originally proposed his model to predict preventive health behaviour, which was later on extended by Kasl and Cobb (1966) to explain sick—role behaviour. More recently, Tanner-Smith (2010) added the dimension of 'contextual constraints' to the health belief model. For example, perceived susceptibility and severity may be high, but if one is struggling with poverty, additional stressors may supersede actions to preserve health.

Some important beliefs (not incorporated in the Health Beliefs Model) that have larger implications for understanding people's reaction to their sickness and subsequent recovery are causal and recovery beliefs: the manner in which people understand and identify the causes of their illness, and beliefs about which factors will contribute to their recovery (Dalal, 1988). A large number of researchers have noted that people suffering from acute or chronic illness develop their own theories about the factors responsible for their illness (Meyerowitz, 1980; Taylor, 1983). People's own theories about the causes of illness include, stress, some virus, physical imbalance, evil spirit, God's will, etc. These causal attributions tell us whether the patients will blame themselves, another person, situational factors or cosmic factors for the problem. For example, if a patient attributes his disease to some evil spirit, he would visit a priest, *ojha, pir* or some witch doctor for the treatment. On the other hand, if a patient attributes his illness to himself (wrong habits or careless-ness), he may have a feeling of guilt, may try to change his own behaviour and would show greater compliance to the treatment regimen.

Consistent with the above position, the psychomedical model does not consider patient as a passive recipient of the treatment but views him or her as an equal partner in the fight against the physical illness. Any treatment involves both the practitioner and the patient, and both need to cooperate in the complex venture. In the case of chronic disease, for example, the experience and knowledge of the patient may be of great value to the practitioners in deciding the future course of action. An ideal patient–practitioner relationship can dramatically enhance the efficacy of treatment and the process of a patient's recovery (Taylor, 2006). The patients who are taught to be aware, optimistic and in con-trol of their lives get well sooner and more completely than passive and helpless patients. The new approach should transform rigid impersonal medical treatment to be more humane, where patient is a partner in search of a suitable cure. Cousins (1979) discovered that a sick person's most desperate need is contact on a personal level with his doctor, and an assurance that things are going to be alright. Furthermore, patients with chronic diseases have many spiritual needs, which remain unat-tended. In a recent study among patients with cancer, a majority (72%) reported that their spiritual needs were supported minimally or not at all by the medical system and 47% felt these were supported minimally or not at all by the religious communities too. This is of importance because spiritual support is associated with better quality of life. It may be difficult for patients to express their spiritual needs (even within close family relationships), and health-care programmes need to address them (Molzahn and Sheilds, 2008). In plural health-care systems prevalent in India, patients feel free to consult a medical doctor for their organic problem and a spiritual healer for their mental and spiritual healing (Joshi, 1988).

An important distinction in the psychomedical approach is made between curing and healing (Dalal, 2010). Curing is removal of the disease, whereas healing implies psychological recovery of patients from that trauma. The emphasis in curing is on restoring physical functioning of the body; healing on the other hand focuses on restoring psychologi-cal health of the patient by bringing changes in beliefs and expectations. A cancer patient might have been medically cured but his anxiety and sense of helplessness may persist for long, at times needing institutional help. In traditional Indian medical system, the distinction between curing and healing is clearly maintained. Even ordinary people maintain this distinction (Joshi, 1988; Kakar, 1982). Joshi (1988) in his study in Central Himalayas discovered that people make a distinction between *bis*, a primary, supernatural and actual cause and *bimari*, a secondary effect for which one gets medical treatment. Thus, when they go to a medical doctor, they talk about physical symptoms, which a doctor can cure. But when the same person goes to a priest, *hakim*, *pir*, *ojha* or *vaid*, he or she follows a different line of causation. They talk about emotional and psychic disorders to remove primary, supernatural and 'actual' causes of the disease. Thus, when a person falls sick the measures for curing and healing are initiated simultaneously. In Indonesia, particularly in Bali, it is one of the responsibilities of a traditional healer to refer a patient to any medical doctor. Consequently, even when cured of the physical ailment, patients return to the same healers for holy water (Sinha, 1988). India, too, has a very rich tradition of healing practices (Dalal, 2010; Kakar, 1982, 2003). The Ayurvedic practitioners do combine healing and curing components of the treatment. The purpose of this chapter is not to discuss them at length, but to drive home a point that the psychomedical model has the potential to take care of both the healing and curing aspects of the treatment by attending to psychological and physical health, respectively. This provides enough scope to incorporate various features of our traditional health-care system in the existing health programmes (Dalal, 2010).

In this respect, the psychomedical approach is more eclectic in nature, where emphasis is on the overall recovery of the patient. The patient is not only successfully treated of a disease but actually feels recovered. The focus is on the person, his or her feelings, anxieties and one's own subjective construction of the illness, which becomes an integral part of the treatment regimen. This approach is thus much closer to the WHO's definition of health as a state of complete physical, mental and social well-being, not merely an absence of a disease.

In fact, bringing a person back to normal health is a challenge not only for medical doctors but also for the family, community, social workers, traditional healers, social scientists, etc. The approach ought to be sufficiently broad-based where healers and specialists from different systems can join hands to bring the person back to good health (Dalal, 2013). A complete model is presented in Chapter 3.

Practical Implications of the Psychomedical Model

The proposed psychomedical model envisions many possibilities of improving health status of people and consequently, improving the quality of the health-care programmes. The model envisages many practical possibilities. This model envisages a more proactive role for social scientists, counsellors, spiritual leaders, traditional health practitioners in planning health-care services. Public health is too serious a matter to be left only in the hands of medical professionals, who have no formal training in handling socio-cultural and psychological aspects of the illness. The health-care system need to be made more broad-based, so that it can handle all the facets of the problem, including public education about health and hygiene. Apart from providing curative services, rural health centres should have been the nucleus of all-round development. To achieve this dream, it is important that social workers, school teachers, religious leaders and even faith healers are closely associated with the activities of the health centres. Indonesian health services have shown the way, where traditional healers are trained to refer serious cases to medical professionals, but these patients come back to the traditional healer for holy water, once they are cured. This system, thus, not only relieves pressure on the medical practitioners, but also takes care of both curing and healing aspects of the disease. Such a system may succeed in Indian conditions. The Government statistics show that India has 5 million traditional practitioners, which include *vaids*, homeopaths, Yunani and other folk health practitioners. These enormous resources have not been systematically utilized by the health planners so far.

The psychomedical model is of much relevance in organizing community health services. A large number of community health programmes have failed in the past because they did not take into consideration local culture, community resources and expectations of the people. A careful understanding of the local community is necessary to mobilize their support and active involvement in health programmes (Dalal, 2010). Early detection, secondary prevention and rehabilitation are the activities that local community can itself take over with minimum training, lessening their dependence on medical services. Such programmes will not only be cost-effective but also easily accessible and acceptable to those who would otherwise go unattended.

2

Health Beliefs and Living with Chronic Diseases

Traditional health-care systems in any culture are mostly based on certain shared beliefs about the world, self and human existence, both in the physical and metaphysical sense. Cultural beliefs provide the necessary framework to define health, to understand the causes of an illness and to decide about the course of treatment. Health beliefs in this sense are part of a broader cultural belief system, which affect the health behaviour of people within a community. Every culture has its characteristic ways of defining health and illness, and recommending the modes of treatment. For example, health beliefs prevalent in the West are based on the assumption of bio-organic causation of diseases, and consequently treatment regimen heavily relies on modern medicines. On the other hand, in many traditional societies of Asia, belief in supernatural causation structures health-related beliefs, choice of treatment alternatives and expectations from health professionals. Thus, in the case of an illness, whereas in the western societies medical hospitals and doctors are visited, in all Asian countries traditional healers are often frequented to deal with physical, mental, interpersonal and existential problems.

Cultural beliefs influence the whole gamut of health-related behaviour. However, this chapter is primarily confined to discussing how these beliefs help people in appraisal and social construction of their illness experience. These cultural beliefs may not play a predominant role in cases of acute and life-threatening diseases where the immediate concern is to save a life, as in the case of heart attack. However, in the case of a long-term disease or disability the concern shifts to bringing changes in one's life to adjust to the demands of the new situation. Family, friends and social network play an important role in shaping a patient's perception of the disease and its implication for his or her life. Most of the patients gradually reconcile to the fact that the chronic disease has become a part of their existence and that cannot be wished away. What a patient believes is more important in such cases where a major responsibility of treatment and care rests on the patient, and how much they will recover depends on their own efforts.

With the increase in life expectancy in recent times, the prevalence of chronic diseases is also on the increase. Of the 36 million global deaths in 2008, 29 million deaths occurred due to non-communicable diseases, which is roughly 63% of the total number of deaths that year. The four main causes of deaths due to chronic diseases are cardiovascular diseases, cancers, diabetes and chronic lung diseases. The burden of these diseases is rising disproportionately among lower income countries and populations. In 2008, nearly 80% of all non-communicable disease occurred in low- and middle-income countries with about 29% of deaths occurring before the age of 60 years (WHO, 2010). Presently, about 70% of the world population above 55 years of age suffers from one or the other chronic diseases and this number is rapidly increasing over the years.

Defining Chronic Disease

Which diseases should be considered as chronic conditions? By definition, chronic diseases are long-lasting diseases, often lasting for the lifetime. The symptoms may not be present all the time, but the prospects of recurrence of the symptoms means that recovery prospects are limited. Second, for such diseases the therapeutic intervention is limited to symptomatic treatment, not complete cure of the disease. Three, because of the long-drawn nature of the disease, people are required to integrate it in their lives. These diseases become part of their existence. The meaning these diseases acquires in one's life largely depend on age, nature of occupations, achievements and responsibilities, and social support one has. Four, in case of chronic diseases there is a good deal of uncertainty about the future course of the disease, its debilitating conditions, and associated physical and psychological complications. The afflicted person is required to comprehend the significance of the chronic diseases in terms of the nature of adjustments that are to be made to live with a disease in the world of healthy. Five, the person suffering from a chronic condition is required to take up major responsibility of managing his/her own disease. The afflicted person is required to identify the symptoms, monitor progress of the disease and control its debilitating side effects. It becomes the responsibility of the people suffering and their families to manage medical, occupational, social and psychological after-effects and to restore one's sense of self-worth and meaning in life. They are not only required to live with the illness but also have to continue participating in every-day life; not as a patient but as a social-being.

Very often in the literature a distinction is made between chronic disease and chronic illness. Kleinman (1978) refers to disease as related to the physical aspect, its physical symptoms, organic malfunctioning, as something going wrong with the person's body. An illness, on the contrary, means a subjective representation of the disease, a psychological experience of being sick. Cassell (1991) also makes a similar kind of distinction between chronic disease and chronic illness. Chronic disease is referred as some disturbance in the structure and functioning of any part, organ or system of the body. While disease is confined to the body, illness was referred to as a disorder in the person's extended system, including family and even community.

Opting in favour of simplification, in this chapter the terms chronic disease and chronic illness are used interchangeably. In the whole discussion, disease or illness is viewed from the patients' point of view. This fact is also acknowledged that a person suffering from a chronic disease cannot be always called a patient, as in the case of bronchitis. People suffering from chronic disease become patient only when their chronic disease becomes acute. It may be noted that a person suffering from a chronic disease may be acutely ill, even in the absence of physical symptoms, as in the case of heart disease. It may be due to the cumulative effect of strain and the anxiety of putting up with a long-term disease. The term patient is thus used here in a very broad sense.

The question of interest here is 'What do people go through while facing a disease of a chronic nature?' The kind of psychological responses people make and the stages they go through depend on many factors. One is the nature of the disease itself. The onset of a disease could be sudden, as in the case of heart attack, or gradual, in which case the patients get sufficient time to deal with the disease. The disease could be life threatening, as cancer, or may go through an acute-chronic cycle, as in asthma. It could be a physically disabling disease, requiring a lot of changes in one's life routine, like arthritis, or demanding more attention and self-care, like diabetes. Some diseases take a heavy toll of one's financial, social and psychological resources, some others are minor nuisances for the person. Again the severity of the disease, their social background, support system and individual dispositions play a crucial role in determining the stages the patients go through in coping with a chronic disease. Most patients eventually recover and both psychologically and physically reach a state of reasonable psychological adjustment, but for about 25% to 30% of patients, the adjustment phase is prolonged and sometimes unsuccessful.

In a large number of cases, when the initial reaction to the diagnosis of chronic disease is that of shock and disbelief, people actively seek disconfirming evidences. People take time to reconcile with the idea that they are suffering from a disease with which they have to live for a long time, maybe for the rest of their lives. They oscillate between hope and despair, and go through extreme mood swings. At a later stage, when a realization dawns that they have to live with the disease, acceptance of the chronic disease comes gradually. People seek more information about the disease and its remedial and palliative aspects. They may like to comprehend its possible implications on their lives. There are active explorations about their own role in containing or preventing the after-effects and integrating the disease within their own lives. People in their endeavour to live with the disease go through the cycles of improvement, remission, relapse and renewed efforts.

Patients with chronic conditions often have to adjust their aspirations, lifestyle and employment. Chronic condition makes them dependent on others socially, economically and even for daily living. They grieve the loss of their healthy state, feel distressed and develop psychiatric disorders, most commonly depression or anxieties. A prospective study of general medical admissions found that 13% of men and 17% of women had an affective disorder (Guthrie, 1996). He further observed that the proportion of patients with conditions such as diabetes or rheumatoid arthritis who have an affective disorder is between 20% and 25%. It can be difficult to diagnose depression in the chronically ill. Physical symptoms such as disturbed sleep, impaired appetite and lack of energy may already exist as a result of their chronic condition. Often, treatment for such a medical condition (for example, the use of steroids) may affect the patient's mood, as may the disease process itself. The functional limitations imposed by the disease may result in 'understandable' distress, and some clinicians find it difficult to conceptualize such distress as a depressive disorder (Powell, 1997). The onset of mental health condition may exacerbate physical symptoms, complicating psychological recovery of people with chronic diseases.

How do people live with chronic diseases is one of the most fascinating and challenging areas of research in psychology. The research in this area has been growing in recent years, though there is still little consistency in the findings that have emerged. There are many reasons for this lack of consistency in the research findings. First, a bulk of research is from the medical perspective, where the emphasis is on the disease, not on the person. The effort is to understand the nature of the disease, to arrive at an accurate diagnosis, and to plan out the treatment procedure. Patients' own perspective and their own perception and feelings are not much investigated. Second, patients' own role in managing the disease is still the least explored. Like the attending doctor, the patient is also actively involved in understanding the disease and trying out various remedial measures. Patients' own beliefs about the illness play an important role in this venture. It is suggested in many studies that patients' own beliefs about their health and treatment regulate their health behaviour to greater extent than the doctors' beliefs or objective medical data. However, there are not many longitudinal studies examining these aspects. Third, the role of cultural factors is relatively ignored in psychological researches in this area. Though there is substantial anthropological and sociological work to highlight cultural differences in health practices and treatment modalities, psychologists have yet to provide an understanding of how these cultural beliefs gets translated into concrete actions. Psychological researches may fall into some pattern if cultural beliefs and their psychological imports are more systematically investigated.

To put it briefly, research focusing on health beliefs should be built on shared understanding about the human nature (Dalal, 2011). First, people are generally actively involved in understanding the meaning of their illness. This understanding is essential to appropriately react to the health crisis. Second, people differ widely in the way they subjectively construct the experience of even very similar illnesses. Their beliefs about the illness and life in general provide the basic inputs for these subjective constructions. Third, these subjective constructions of the illness in terms of their meaning, causes and control influence their recovery (or adjustment) significantly, at times more significantly than the nature of the disease. Fourth, people are motivated to make efforts to recover from the crisis situation. In fact, it is assumed that the efforts to recover begin with the onset of the chronic disease itself. Fifth, people are not only motivated but also possess a self-curing mechanism. In the crisis situation, this mechanism gets activated and people in few instances need institutional support to deal with the psychological crisis. People not only recover or successfully adjust but also learn to be more resourceful in facing a similar crisis in future. Sixth, people can be helped and trained to cope with the adversities by bringing appropriate changes in their own beliefs and attitudes.

Plurality of the Health-care Systems

One important factor that makes it imperative to study the health beliefs of the patients is the multiple modalities of treatments existing in all traditional societies of Asia. Each system has its own assumptions about health, its causes and the curative mode. Decision about the treatment modality greatly depends on the kind of beliefs the patients and their social support network have about the illness.

Working primarily in the Asian region, Kleinman (1978) classified health-care systems in traditional societies in three main sectors. These are the popular sector, the folk sector and the professional sector. Each sector has its own mode of interpreting and treating an illness, and defining the role of the healer and the patients.

The popular sector: This is the most informal, non-professional mode of health care. This kind of therapeutic advice is provided without any payment to social network, religious institutions and self-help groups. The treatment is generally provided at home where family provides the basic health care. It is estimated that about 70% to 90% of health care takes place within this sector. The health practices in this sector are primarily guided by the communities' own beliefs about healthy way to drink, eat, sleep, work, etc. and practices, such as home-made remedies, proper diet and care to maintain good health.

The folk sector: Trained informally, or through apprenticeship, some people in society specialize in healing people suffering from different ailments, both physical and mental. There are diverse types of folk healers—from purely shamans and spiritual healers to technical experts like herbalists, bone-setters and midwives. These folk healers belong to the same community, share the basic cultural values and world views, including beliefs about the causes, significance and treatment of ill health. Most of these systems have divinity as basic to their practice and often the practitioners are presumed to possess some divine powers. These folk healers are mostly holistic in their approach and involve the family, other community members and supernatural entities in the treatment procedure.

The professional sector: In the original sense this refers to modern western medicine. These include the medical personnel formally trained and legally permitted to deal with patients. This category also includes the paramedical staff. However, as Kleinman noted, in some traditional medical systems such as Ayurveda, Unani, homeopathy, acupuncture practitioners are trained in the professional schools. These medical systems also come in this category. It can be mentioned here that in most of the Asian and African countries western medicine is accessible to only a small section of the society and people still subscribe to these traditional systems. In India, for example, western medical care is available to less than 8% of the population.

It is not that people always stick to only one sector of treatment. On the contrary, people alternate or try more than one mode of treatment at the same time. People who suffer a disease often resort to different modes of treatment, within or across all three sectors, as they may really not know what will really work in their case. However, in recent years with wider reach of medical facilities more people are seeking medical care, but in the process they are also experiencing the limitations of drug and surgical therapies.

Meaning of Health Belief

Clearly patients' response to chronic conditions will depend on their lager belief system within which they understand various life events. Such beliefs are the basis of our thoughts and understanding of the world we live in. They provide the basis for decision and actions we take in everyday life. These beliefs we acquire in social interactional process and are sustained because of their functional value. These beliefs cannot be viewed in isolation but they serve as integrated and cohesive constituents of a larger belief system pertaining to all domains of life. Cultural and social milieu creates the context for formation, change and maintenance of these beliefs, and also for interpreting the experiential world we live in. Indigenous health beliefs, in this sense, need to be examined as part of the belief system of a society.

Beliefs can be understood as shared and assumed truths within a cultural set-up. Beliefs are thus taken as propositions that are considered to be correct and the basis of social interaction. Beliefs are part of our understanding of the world we live in, the people we are, and explanations of happenings. We imbibe many beliefs in the course of growing up in a family and culture. They are part of our consciousness, guiding our thoughts and actions. Beliefs here do not refer to subconscious thoughts, or a mental activity occurring below the threshold of consciousness. When a person owns a belief, he or she consciously accepts its meaning and implication. The degree of valence with which one owns a belief can vary from mild acceptance to confident certainty. Beliefs require conscious acceptance. Furthermore, beliefs may vary in terms of their complexity, centrality and flexibility, as they implicate everyday life of the people.

Taken from this perspective, beliefs lie in the grey area between assumption and knowledge (Walker, 2006). At one extreme they can be termed as dogmas or delusions; in milder form they are termed as faith, convictions, superstitions and misconceptions. *Belief* and *faith* overlaps, both accept the phenomenon *a priori*. However, the rational presumption that often lies behind *belief* is wholly lacking in *faith*. One cannot argue with a faith; it simply *is*. We try to anchor our beliefs in some kind of proof. It may be anchored in some authority, logic or personal observation. It could be mediated through some chain of information, the source of which one can rely on. Religion is one of the most potent sources of beliefs, as is science.

Health beliefs of Indian people are in many ways distinct from the health beliefs of people in western societies. Singh (2011) has examined many such cultural beliefs of the Indian heart patients. Many of these illness beliefs are product of age-old customs, traditions, rituals, mythologies and spiritual texts. These beliefs have evolved over a long history. Some characteristic features of these beliefs can be identified (Dalal, 2011). One, these health beliefs seldom stand independent of the other indigenous beliefs. They are intricately weaved into the other community beliefs. From the ontological standpoint, health is integral to the very fact of living. Health from the Indian perspective is thus seen as part of the general well-being of the individual. It is contended that individual well-being is also contingent on happiness and well-being of others, including well-being of other living beings. Two, traditional health beliefs are part of the sacred. Faith, fear and reverence are the hallmarks of indigenous health beliefs. They are part of the beliefs people have about life and death. Gods, spirits and ancestors are taken as important agencies—causing health crises, as well as triggering recovery process. Three, Indian health beliefs have positive connotation; they are characterized by hope and positivism. This positivism is evident in the way people construe the meaning of their health and well-being and deal with illness incidences. Belief in the theory of karma, for example, seems to facilitate acceptance of tragic life events and help in retaining hopes. Four, people go to the same healer for their health problems, as well as for other wide-ranging problems they face in personal life, including those of business loss or marital discord. People do not make a clear distinction between physical, social and moral problems.

Functional Nature of Health Beliefs

Beliefs influence human health implicitly and explicitly in various ways. The human mind converts beliefs and expectations into biochemical realities. The mechanisms that link beliefs to the bodily processes are still not very clear. Most of the evidences are anecdotal suggesting that these works, but no direct linkages have yet been established. Perhaps the most compelling evidence is provided by the placebo studies. It is observed in a large number of studies that anticipation of physical effects as outcomes of medication placebos bring about actual physical changes. In a study, Fielding et al. (1983) reported that patients were expected to experience hair loss from chemotherapy, but 30% patients who were on placebo instead of chemotherapy suffered hair loss, which was to the same extent as the chemotherapy group. As argued by Radley (1994) where doctors and patients subscribe to the same beliefs strongly and where there is greater faith in doctors, placebos will have more therapeutic powers.

Expectations work varied ways. One related phenomenon 'anniversary effect' signifies that people are more likely to die around important dates in their lives. Phillips et al. (1992) surveyed the records of over 2 million people. It revealed that women are more likely to die within a week after their birthdays; men peak just before their birthday. The interpretation was that women are more likely to believe that birthdays are occasions to celebrate and meet friends and relatives; whereas for men it is a time to take stock of their accomplishments, which they often dread.

Lazarus (1993, 2000) has talked about 'healthy illusions'—the beliefs that make life liveable. Such beliefs (like, I am a good person) are essential to lead a healthy life. Such self-serving illusions include illusion of well-being, illusion of personal control, unrealistic optimism, etc. Such illusions have positivity bias and are associated with subjective well-being. Taylor and Brown (1994) have discussed some of the important functions that healthy illusions serve for people. First, they provide explanations as to why do people fall sick. It is important to have an explanation, no matter how aversive it is to make life events predictable. It helps people in having mental preparations to face the hard truth. Second, beliefs about the causes of illness help people in deciding about the kind of treatment to be sought. People postpone decisions regarding the alternative medicine to be sought till they are sure about the causality. Third, beliefs play an important role in building hopes and expectations, which trigger the healing mechanism of the body. People who expect to die on the operation table often fail the surgery. Beliefs help people in reintegrating within the culture they come from. Cultural beliefs help find meaning in their suffering. Dalal (2011) has discussed cultural beliefs about self and health in India, which have such positivity bias and thus implicates recovery from chronic diseases.

Indian Perspective on Disease and Suffering

Suffering is believed to be a universal characteristic of the human condition though its causality is understood in different ways in different cultures. In Hindu and Buddhist traditions, it is viewed as a mental state, a personal experience (Miri, 1976). The personal experience of falling ill is subsumed within the holistic conception of well-being and suffering. Conversely, as the sage Vedavyasa says in his commentary on Patanjali's Yoga Sutra (2.15), suffering is like a disease and yoga is like the medicine for its removal (as quoted by Paranjpe, 1984). Thus, though traditional medicine and healing systems pay attention to physical pain, they often lay their emphasis on removal of suffering in its holistic sense.

The distinctiveness of the Indian approach lies in trying to eliminate the root causes of the problem, and thereby focusing on the *sufferer* rather than on the *suffering*. In the Samkhya, as well as in many other classical philosophical systems of India, the thrust of inquiry is more on finding out who is it that experiences pleasure and pain, than on what is being experienced (Paranjpe, 1998). The Ayurvedic theory of medicine is consistent with this viewpoint and insists that medicine should target the person rather than the disease. The person in wholeness is called the 'asylum' of disease and constitutes the main subject of medicine (Kakar, 1982). The Ayurvedic science thus focuses on the knowledge of the patient's present mental state and his more enduring personality traits, which should be supplemented with gaining a thorough familiarity with his familial, social, geographical and cultural contexts. It takes into consideration different levels of human existence: physical, mental, social and metaphysical and a harmony among these different levels of existence.

The main treatise of the Sankhya system, *Sankhya Karika* has provided the most exhaustive understanding of the causes of suffering and disease. The three different sets of factors are presumed to cause suffering. These are material factors (*adhibhautika*), sorcery (*adhidaivika*) and self (*adhyatmika*). Self refers to both bodily and mental causes. The physical causes include bodily conditions as well as social and environmental factors, which adversely affect health conditions. Sorcery refers to spirits, demons and deities that can be taken care of by offering prayers, chanting mantras, wearing amulets and visiting spiritual healers. The bodily conditions of disease were caused by imbalances of the body. The bodily conditions of disease are supposed to be caused by imbalance of three life energies (*tridoshas*) and could be alleviated by taking medicine and regulating diet. From the Sankhya viewpoint, mental suffering consists of affective reactions like greed, envy, lust, etc. The complete annihilation of suffering is thus possible when all the causes of suffering are removed (Paranjpe, 1998, 2006). In this endeavour not only physicians, but family, friends, society and traditional healers also are presumed to play an important role. The vast variety of healing systems practiced in India work on these basic premises.

Coping with Chronic Diseases

In the light of the above discussion, it should now be possible for us to explore more systematically how people react and put up with a disease at its different stages? How health beliefs get translated into relevant health behaviour? In the following presentation, these questions will be dealt with in greater detail.

Onset of an Illness

When do people realize that they are chronically sick? In some instances like coronary heart disease, the impinging reality leaves no scope for thinking otherwise. However, in most of the other instances it takes quite long for patients to reconcile with the fact that they are chronically sick. People tend to believe, even in the face of hard evidences to the contrary, that they will be fully cured. When the disease is diagnosed as chronic, there is a tendency to explore the possibility of an error in the diagnosis. People are very susceptible at this stage to suggestions that the disease is curable. Even patients at the advanced stage of cancer are found to be hopeful of complete cure (Kubler-Ross, 1975).

In the Indian setting, it is generally not during the routine check-up that the disease is detected. When people observe some unusual symptoms or bodily changes, they confide it to their close relatives and friend, who help in interpreting the symptoms to arrive at a naïve diagnosis (Singh, 1987). These are the people in close social network who provide initial interpretations about the possible implications of the symptoms. Those who appraise the illness as still at the initial stage may try domestic remedies. In quite a number of cases, formal medical check-up does not take place to arrive at a diagnosis. There is a greater degree of reliance on the diagnosis made by elders, priests and paramedical personnel (Banerjee, 1986).

Once a diagnosis of the chronic disease dawns upon the patient, the immediate crisis reaction may be that of fear and anxiety. The patient is uncertain as to how to handle the anxiety. An easy way out is to refuse to accept the diagnosis or to delink symptoms from the illness, and thus unconsciously blocks any cognizance of the illness. This state, however, cannot last long, as the increasing evidence and everyday inconvenience usually makes it difficult for the patient to sweep the hard realities of their health under the rug. The other option for the patients is to accept the diagnosis but resort to other ego-defence mechanisms such as rationalization, compartmentalization, isolation, displacement, projection and the like. These patients belittle the significance of the symptoms, delay seeking medical care, or fail to comply with the treatment regimen and the rehabilitation programme. One such example is of heart patients who oftentimes procrastinate in seeking diagnosis, and thereby jeopardize their chances of survival.

At some stage when the patients come to terms with realities a new phase of crisis begins. The acceptance of a diagnosis of chronic disease triggers several major worries. One needs to ascertain as to how much functioning will be impaired by the illness? How can it be integrated with their lives in the long-term perspective? What kind of adjustments they would be required to make in their occupational and social life? Generally, patients get enough time to ponder over the illness and its consequences, test their naïve theories of illness and recovery, and form some stable opinion about the causes of the illness and about appropriate coping strategies. These inquisitive exercises, which Lazarus (1981) has called secondary appraisal, are essential to clear some of the mist shrouding the illness.

Subjective Meaning of an Illness

People assign meaning to their illness in many different ways. As pointed out by a medical sociologist (Parson, 1972), the sick role is necessarily socially deviant and society will permit it only after the doctor legitimizes the patient's need, both to regress and accept the sick condition. Psychologists, however, take a different viewpoint. Herzlich's (1973) empirical study focused on social psychological meaning and implications of health and illness as stages of being. The respondents regarded illness as an intrusion, an external imposition, which renders a person passive and powerless. Herzlich observed that when people face an illness, particularly a long-term one, their self-perceptions are blurred. To regain some sense of self-sensibility, they need to make sense out of their illness. Sometimes the need to understand the illness is so compelling that it actually overshadows the desire to be cured.

Such understanding of the meaning of illness includes beliefs about the symptoms, causes, consequences, cures and duration of illness are thought to be derived from personal experiences with illness, support group, health professional and social networks. Two important aspects of illness perceptions are that patients' beliefs about their condition are often at variance from those who are treating them, and secondly, patients' perceptions vary widely, even in patients with the same medical condition (Petrie et al., 2007). Many studies have investigated the relationships between illness perceptions and outcomes in different patient populations. A meta-analysis of 45 empirical studies among patients with various medical conditions, demonstrated that perceptions that the illness was curable/controllable were significantly and positively related to the adaptive outcomes of psychological well-being, social functioning and vitality, and negatively related to psychological distress and disease state. Conversely, perceptions of illness consequences, timeline and identity exhibited significant, negative relationships with psychological well-being, role, and social functioning and vitality (Hagger and Orbell, 2003; Leventhal and Benyamini, 1997). In 1986, Turk et al. developed a 45-item Implicit Models of Illness Questionnaire (IMIQ), which includes questions assessing the components of illness representations. They identified a four-factor structure using this scale: seriousness, personal responsibility, controllability and changeability.

Clearly, the meaningful understanding that a sick person seeks is not limited to the medical explanations of one's sickness. Patients extend their formulations to embrace the social, psychological implications for themselves and their family. This view is contrary to the view held by psychoanalysts who regard illness as 'motivated' (Lipowski, 1983). The cognitive view advocated here considers it unlikely that many people actively seek illness. It is possible that some patients may impart neurotic meaning to it, for example, they may view illness as a punishment or as an escape from the rigor of life.

Lipowski (1978) also examined in greater detail the different meanings, which people assign to their illness. These are illness as a challenge (insightful acceptance), illness as an enemy, illness as punishment, illness as weakness, illness as relief, illness as a strategy (as a means), illness as an irreparable loss and damage, and illness as value. The meaning that a person assigns to his or her illness is predominantly conscious, but at time may be unconscious, influencing one's emotional and motivational response to the disease. Lipowski further suggested the different emotional reactions and coping strategies associated with these meanings. Schussler (1992) studying patients with chronic problems found overall support for the illness concepts of Lipowski. For example, it was found that patients who viewed their disease as a challenge showed no anxiety and depression and were emotionally stable, whereas those who viewed their disease as an enemy or as a punishment were on the other end of the same continuum. It is, however, an open question as to how those who view their illness as a punishment from God will emotionally react to their illness.

Beliefs about Personal Control

Belief in personal control is defined by most of the theorists as a belief that one has at one's disposal, a response that can influence the aversiveness of an event. It is argued that the belief in personal control is integral to self-concept and self-esteem, constituting a fundamental psychological state. Fighting a chronic disease and long-term hospitalization quite often undermines one's sense of personal control and a sense of helplessness pervades. To have an effective coping, it is essential that people regain some amount of control. Most of the theories of personal control predict that feeling of control reduces the experience of stress; it helps people cope with unavoidable, unpleasant events and enable them to live a better life. Moreover, these theories recognize that control does not need to be exercised for it to be effective and it does not even need to be real for it to have desired effects.

Building on the typologies suggested by Averill (1973) and Miller and Norman (1979), Thompson (1981) developed a four-fold typology of perceived controllability: behavioural, cognitive, information and retrospective. People can control the course of their illness in many ways. Thompson (1981) identified five types of control beliefs, which patients can exercise in a crisis situation. One is *behavioural control*, which is the belief in one's ability to take some steps to reduce the intensity of the illness, can reduce its frequency, or can alter its timing and duration. Patients believe that by taking appropriate actions, negative consequences of the prolonged sickness can be averted. To be effective, behavioural control need not be real, the belief that one can take steps to control one's illness is sufficient to reduce distress. Second is *cognitive control*, which is the availability of some cognitive skills to think differently about the illness. For example, a hospitalized patient about to undergo a painful diagnostic medical procedure may be instructed to focus on the benefits of the procedure rather than on the current discomfort. *Decision control* is the belief in the ability to make decisions about the future course of action. The patients who believed that they have options to choose from are capable of making their own decisions. The fourth is *information control*, which is a sense of control achieved when one acquires sufficient information about the obnoxious event itself. A patient awaiting surgery, for example, may have all post-operative side effects carefully explained, so that when they occur, it will not be distressing. The fifth is *retrospective control*, a term coined by Thompson, to refer to the belief that the event that just occurred was controllable, thereby implying that its reoccurrence can be controlled in future. He stated that the kind of control exercised would depend on the appraisal of the potentially stressful event by the individual.

Another important theory was proposed by Rothbaum et al. (1982). Their two-process model of perceived control claimed that people attempt to gain control not only by bringing the environment into line with their wishes (primary control) but also by bringing themselves into line with environmental forces (secondary control). According to Rothbaum et al., four manifestations of secondary control (changing oneself) are (i) predictive control by attributing the event to severely limited ability, thus guarding oneself against future disappointment; (ii) attribution to luck, which can lead to illusory control; this occurs when luck is construed as a personal characteristic; (iii) vicarious control, when the individual identifies him or herself with the powerful others (God or a leader); (iv) interpretive control, in which the individual seeks to understand and derive meaning from the otherwise uncontrollable events in order to accept them. About 27 years later, Rothbaum et al. (2009) tested and validated their model for its contemporary relevance taking patients suffering from depression.

Since personal control is believed to be effective in dealing with everyday events as well as health-related events, people under some circumstances exaggerate the degree of control they have, in situations that are chance happenings, thus developing what Langer (1975) called an 'illusion of control'. This illusion of control is very frequently manifested in choosing auspicious occasions such as 'lucky' numbers in buying a lottery ticket, playing cricket with a lucky bat, etc. In many instances, this illusion of control is healthy in the sense that people strive hard to prevent an undesirable outcome. But it may greatly aggravate the stress if a tragic event shatters this illusion. Beliefs of more personal control, less impact of the illness and its treatment, and less concern were the most important contributors to perceived autonomy and self-esteem in case of chronic kidney patients (Jansen et al., 2010).

In recent years, the basic assumptions of theories of perceived controllability that people seek control and that the control is desirable are questioned. Carver et al. (2000) argued that perceived control is salient to the extent it enhances the expectation of recovery. Conducting a study on cancer patients, they showed that expectation of remaining cancer-free was a good predictor of distress, but perceived control over the disease was not. As pointed out by Taylor (1984), 'control is a double-edged sword', it is beneficial in some circumstances and not under others; it is beneficial for some people and not for others; it may work in one cultural set-up and fail in the other.

It is now argued that people are often willing to give up control depending on their understanding of the tragic circumstances, rather than seeking more personal control. Misra (1994) argued that the theory of personal control needs to be viewed from a larger cross-cultural perspective. According to Misra, the idea of control in the Indian scripture is seen in the framework of consciousness, harmony and interrelatedness, not from the individual perspective. Personal control is considered to be an illusion in an interconnected world and the human suffering is needed to be seen from a larger cosmic perspective. In fact, sense of personal (ego) control is viewed as a major causative factor in precipitating pain and suffering. Studies have revealed the chaos and mental health problem which this cultural ideal of sense of personal control has caused in the West (Schwartz, 2000). Giving up the sense of personal control and accepting the destiny is many times prescribed as the remedy for alleviation of the suffering one is going through. The message of the Gita that one has control over the efforts one can make, not on the outcome can help in alleviating pain and suffering (Bhawuk, 2012). One has to learn what one can control and what one cannot. Surrender and 'letting go' are the other concepts, which need to be critically examined for their role in dealing with health- and illness-related issues.

Health Beliefs and Affective Reactions

A wide variety of reactions are observed when people are told about the diagnosis of a chronic illness. Quite often, the initial reaction is that of denial or disbelief, which averts the onset of any emotional crisis. Denial also gives some time to adjust to the impinging reality. Other typical reactions are of high anxiety and emotional disturbance, clouding clear thinking. On the other hand, there are people who accept the diagnosis rather stoically. Chronic illness is something people have to live with, and they have to make long-term alterations in their lifestyle. There could be wide fluctuations in the mood of patients with changes in their physical conditions and nature of disability. Pain and discomfort are other factors influencing the affective state. Many of these affective reactions may be transitory or of diffused kind, whereas other reactions are specific to the appraisal of the symptoms. Broadly speaking, affective reactions could be of two types—a general response to the situation like fear, sadness, unpleasantness, anxiety, etc., and those which are belief dependent. The belief-related affects are often very specific reactions, based on causal beliefs and control the appraisal of the situation. Such affective reactions are those of anger, depression, disappointment, pity, etc.

Studies have been done to establish linkages between affective reactions to an undesirable life condition, and causal and control-related beliefs. Causal appraisal gives rise to a qualitative distinction among the feelings. Weiner (1985) found that in the case of giving help, lack of effort on the part of the help seeker aroused anger, whereas physical disability led to aroused feeling of pity. Dalal and Tripathi (1987) in a study of help-seeking behaviour found the linkages between control beliefs (situation controllable or uncontrollable) and affective reactions stable and reversible. Some attribution–affect linkages found in their two experimental studies were uncontrollable sympathy, controllable anger and dislike.

The onset of a chronic illness and subsequent hospitalization result in more frequent feelings of anxiety, depression, suppressed anger and helplessness (Westbrook and Viney, 1982). In an Indian study by Agrawal and Dalal (1993), the dominant affective reactions found in hospitalized patients were helplessness, depression and metaphysical rationalization. There were some gender differences: female patients showed greater anger and anxiety, whereas male patients more often engaged in disengagement and rationalization. It was also noted that anger was the least frequent reaction. In a study by Kohli (1992) on cancer patients, evidence of anger response was very low. There is a greater degree of acceptance and rationalization in terms of the theory of Karma, where people look for justification in their own wrongdoing in their previous births. Higher attribution to metaphysical factors probably explains why Indian patients are low on anger reaction.

It seems that the feeling more often expressed in response to loss of control is that of helplessness. People show acute helplessness when they feel a loss of control in a tragic situation. When all previously acquired behaviour skills fail to yield any desirable results and the patients start doubting their own ability to exercise any control, then the feeling of helplessness overtakes.

The feeling reported most frequently in the cases of chronic illnesses is that of depression. Depression is characterized by a dejected mood, loss of desire to do things, general tiredness and inability to concentrate. A depressed person may think that nothing can be done to change the undesirable life conditions. Like anger and helplessness, the feeling of depression sets in at a later stage of the chronic illness. During the initial phase of the illness, the patients may be too pre-occupied with diagnostic hospital procedure to feel depressed. The feeling surfaces at a later stage when the patient has tried many treatments unsuccessfully and now has to cope with a host of new problems, related to adjustment in his day-to-day living. Many researchers suggest that the emotional reaction of depression is beneficial in a sense that it is preparatory to the later adjustments that must be made as a consequence of the illness. However, acute or prolonged depression is pathological.

Compliance with Treatment Regimen

In a chronic illness the treatment is long-drawn, sometimes lifelong, and its discontinuation at any stage may be hazardous. Second, in a chronic illness the onus of adhering to the treatment largely depends on the patient himself or herself, once he or she is out of the critical phase. In diabetes and arthritis, for example, patients are expected to monitor their physical condition, follow the treatment regimen and take necessary precautions. Same is the case with heart patients, where any neglect may be fatal at times. Patients' role in following the treatment regimen thus seems crucial in chronic illness.

Notwithstanding, universally, lack of compliance seems more a rule than exception. WHO (2003) inferred that more than 50% of the patients do not take prescribed medication in accordance with the instructions. Thus even in situations where proper medical care is available, compliance is still a problem. The social characteristics of the patients such as age, gender and education were found to be poor predictors of compliance, though a high correlation was found between characteristics of the treatment regimen and nature of patient doctor relationship.

Rosenstock's (1966, 1974) health belief model originally developed to predict preventive health behaviour, was later extended to account for compliance to the treatment regimen. In this health belief model, the perception of threat to health is the most crucial factor. The perceived threat of the disease is determined by two considerations: perceived threat of the disease one is suffering from, or could suffer from, and perceived vulnerability to the illness and its consequences. For example, a diabetic would first assess his condition as severe or mild and would think about its possible consequences for his life adjustments, before he perceives diabetes as a threat.

However, this perception of threat is not sufficient to engage in health-care behaviour. One important factor is the belief that a particular health-related activity will protect oneself from the threat. The second factor in the model, which will determine health behaviour, is the perceived cost and benefit of compliance. In order to comply, the patient must believe that the recommended regimen will be effective and the accrued benefits will offset the cost, such as discomfort, side effects and other negative aspects. According to the health belief model, to initiate or sustain any treatment regimen, the patient waits for some cues so as to make him/her aware of the potential consequences. Internal cues are very important in this context.

The health belief model is tested taking various chronic illnesses, and is found useful in predicting compliance. Where an illness is diagnosed and a course of treatment recommended, the patients' perception of the threat in terms of symptoms and future consequences becomes crucial. It is in relation to this threat that possible actions and their costs can be evaluated. Becker and Maiman (1975) and Kirscht (1983) reviewed the literature on patient compliance from the point of view of the health belief model. The model has been applied in the studies of compliance to hypertensive regimen (Becker et al., 1977) and cardiac care of rural population (Leight, 2003). There are now a number of studies that do not support the health belief model particularly when unhealthy behaviour is strongly habitual, like cigarette smoking or deeply rooted in the local culture, or where chronic disease is already set in (Rawlett, 2011; Tanner-Smith, 2010).

Attempts have been made in the past to enhance compliance through systematic changes in health attitudes and beliefs. Tagliacozzo and others (1984) examined the role of information in compliance behaviour. To the experimental group, a special nurse gave detailed instructions about various aspects of the disease, whereas the control group received regular medical care. There was no effect of instructions. However, the factors found in that study having the significant impact were duration of illness, multiple illnesses, high anxiety, favourable attitude towards the clinic and the doctor, and perceived severity of illness. It appears that any information, which is general and abstract does not result in compliance.

It was observed in many studies that those patients who show helplessness and depression also show poor compliance. Some interventions using attributional concepts have tried to inculcate a sense of self-efficacy and self-control. One such study was conducted by Chambliss and Murray (1979). In their study, the subjects who were inclined to give up smoking were given a placebo capsule to complement their efforts at self-control. The placebo was described as increasing, decreasing or having no effect on the symptoms of withdrawal. In the second phase of the study, half of the subjects were told that the drug was inactive and that they had reduced their smoking through their own efforts, while the rest of the subjects were not debriefed at all. The debriefed group, and in particular those with an internal locus of control, went on to reduce their smoking by a significantly greater amount than the others. Colletti and Kopel (1979) also reported that the more the subjects attributed their improvement to their own efforts, the less they were smoking one year later. Sonney and Janoff (1982) gave their obese patients a choice between two weight loss programmes, one emphasizing self-control and another external control by the therapist. Both programmes were equally effective during the treatment period, but the self-control group maintained better progress, as found in the follow-up interview.

Living with Chronic Illness

Learning to live with any long-term adversity is always problematic. How people will cope with their chronic condition will depend on the nature of illness, its severity and socio-psychological resources, which people have to deal with. The most difficult initial problem is to accept the fact that one has to live with the chronic disease they are suffering from. In spite of medical confirmation, people find it hard to accept it as a reality of their life. As discussed earlier, many people continue in the denial mode, keep seeking one or the other course of treatment and repeated failures make them feel worse. The more time they take to reconcile with the reality, the more complicated the process of readjusting in life becomes.

Once the diagnosis of chronic illness is accepted and patients have reconciled to the fact that they have to live with it, the spotlight shifts on efforts to integrate the illness in the patients' lives. The concern is how to go about that and how soon can patients be brought back to their usual life routine. In a large number of cases, a major readjustment is required. The self-management of chronic illness is characterized by taking responsibilities regarding medication use and lifestyle changes, and taking steps to prevent long-term complications.

Much would depend on the extent of physical impairment due to the illness. Physical problems engendered by the illness range widely. Breathlessness associated with asthma, metabolic changes in diabetic patients, motor coordination problems in spinal cord injury cases, and impaired body limb movement associated with arthritis are a few examples of the physical problems. There may be psychological problems, such as loss of memory in epilepsy, for example, with which patients are required to put up with.

In many chronic illnesses, such as arthritis, pain is the most disturbing consequence. Sometimes treatment of the disease produces chronic pain and discomfort, which by itself poses a management problem. The chronic pain in many instances has greater debilitating effects than the illness itself. Even though it may have a physiological basis, pain is basically a psychological experience. For example, pain can be minimal when attention is distracted but when attention is focused on the pain, the pain experience is heightened. Sternbach (1978) had reported that pain tends to increase as the anxiety level of the person increases. There is considerable research evidence showing that the degree of pain and level of distress that people experience largely depends on the labels and cognitions that are applied to the physical state. Persistent, unrelenting pain and stress often leads to uncertainty and anxiety, which many patients and their families find hard to cope with. People have to frequently resort to taking painkillers, which has its own implications.

Chronic disease affects not only the patients, their families too have to go through major changes in their life conditions. They are needed to mobilize their financial, social and community resources to deal with impending crises. If the person is earning member of the family then chronic condition results in financial crisis as well. It is thus not uncommon for patients and family members to have prolonged periods of worries about the effect the illness on their lives. On the part of the patient worries include physical symptoms, such as difficulty breathing, headache, lack of mobility and body pain. Psychological symptoms of anxiety, such as fear of what will happen, include worrying about who will care for them, and how the illness will progress. What one feels and deals with accompanying emotions can affect one's ability to cope with a long-term chronic condition.

Most of the chronic illness episodes are managed within family set-up. Barring the acute phase of the chronic illness when the patient may need hospitalization, it is the extended and close family, which takes care of the health regimen of the suffering member. Family support is crucial for medical and psychosocial recovery of the person. Though as many studies show, Indian families are overindulging and overprotective, their support is considered crucial to bring the person back to normal routine (Chadda and Deb, 2013).

In chronic illnesses, physical rehabilitation is integral to the treatment procedure itself. According to Taylor (2006), physical rehabilitation of chronically ill patients typically involves several goals: to help them use their body as much as possible, to sensitize patients about the physical changes and reality, and to develop new management skills.

Quite often patients are required to read bodily signals about the onset of the crisis, take precautionary measures, administer medicine, etc. Any comprehensive physical rehabilitation programme must pertain to all or most of these goals. The task is certainly challenging.

In the long term, an even more challenging task is that of psychosocial rehabilitation. Social support and patients' own internal resources are crucial factors in successful long-term coping with the chronic disease. The psychosocial rehabilitation of the patient does not follow a predetermined course; rather there are many ups and downs and uncertainties, which keep cropping up from time to time. Much of the successful rehabilitation depends on patients' positive interaction with people in their socio-cultural milieu. Fortunately, most of the patients show an impressive ability to cope with adverse life conditions. Many of the survival strivings are built-in in the human nature, which are activated whenever survival is endangered. Thus, very few patients need professional help to get rehabilitated (Taylor, 1983).

The phenomenon that facilitates the task of rehabilitation is, what Rosenbaum (1983) termed 'learned resourcefulness'. Learned resourcefulness refers to an acquired repertoire of self-regulated internal responses, such as emotions, pain and cognitions (Rosenbaum, 1983; Rosenbaum and Ben-Ari, 1987). The conditions that activate the self-regulatory process are similar to those that are recognized as stress conditions. In the condition of prolonged stress due to chronic illness, people gradually acquire a large response repertoire to cope successfully. In many instances, it is observed that psychological adjustment or existence is even better than the one prior to the illness.

Against this background, the emphasis of any rehabilitation programme should be to provide an opportunity wherein a patient can learn to be resourceful, that is, acquire self-regulatory skills to live with the illness. Perhaps the important question is how can one learn to be resourceful? Meichenbaum (1977, 1975) developed a stress inoculation programme for this purpose. The major components of the stress inoculation programme are (1) self-monitoring of maladaptive thoughts, images, feelings and behaviours; (2) training in cognitive and behavioural skills, which enable them to cope effectively with stress, and (3) emotion regulation. Meichenbaum argues that those who have acquired these skills develop a sense of learned resourcefulness. It is assumed that without any formal training these behaviours are acquired in different degrees by most of the patients. These behavioural and cognitive skills facilitate the process of rehabilitation. Furthermore, it is suggested here that those who are able to help themselves (highly resourceful persons) will be most helped by others. Those who are unable to help themselves are likely to deplete their social resources by their highly socially dependent behaviour (Monroe and Steiner, 1986; Wortman and Lehman, 1985).

Consistent with this ideology, many self-help programmes are evolved in recent years. The basic philosophy behind self-help is that people who are suffering from similar illnesses can provide mutual support, understanding and information for successful adjustment. It is generally observed that patients tend to bring needed changes in their health habits through sharing experiences with others in the same plight. In a typical self-help programme, people with common illnesses are brought together and often with the help of a counsellor, they attempt to solve their problems collectively. A self-help group emphasizes face-to-face social interaction and assumes personal responsibility on the part of the members. These people come together for mutual assistance in satisfying a common need, that is, overcoming a common handicap or life-disrupting problem, and bringing about desired social and personal changes (Katz and Bender, 1976). In these self-help groups, the patients not only learn the skills to help themselves but also help those who face similar crisis. Borne et al. (1986) reviewed a large number of studies to examine the efficacy of self-help groups of cancer patients. They found positive results in almost all the studies reviewed, that is, improvement in terms of general health perception and reduction in negative feelings.

The mutual support among fellow patients is a widely observed phenomenon. These patients come in contact with each other when they are in-patient in the same hospital ward or visiting the same doctor. Kakar (2003) has described many social and religious institutions in India, which are a common meeting ground for patients and their relatives. Though their functioning is loosely structured and quite informal, they do serve the purpose. At the other extremity, as in the West, contact among fellow patients may be part of a highly structured intervention programme, which is initiated in the hospital. There seems to be enough scope to develop various self-help types of interventions to alleviate the suffering of chronic patients and to accelerate their rehabilitation.

3

Development of an Attributional Model of Psychological Recovery

Two conclusions can be drawn from the preceding chapters. One, cultural beliefs play an important role in providing meaning to the experience of a chronic disease, enabling one to make necessary adjustments in one's life. People derive a meaningful understanding of the disease they are suffering from by sharing their experiences with other people in their social group who generally come from the same cultural background. Two, embedded in the cultural beliefs are the beliefs related to cause and recovery, the factors to which people causally attribute their disease and subsequent recovery. Such causal and recovery beliefs are closely linked with affective and behavioural reactions to the disease, as also with the physical recovery.

However, the research literature is still quite vague about the manner in which causal and recovery beliefs affect psychological recovery of patients. A large number of variables could be mediating between an individual's causal attributions and subsequent recovery, which need to be identified. Why some people recover and others don't in similar circumstances? It appears that though causal beliefs are extensively investigated in numerous studies, their implications for recovery are not sufficiently understood. It is important to examine how causal explanations of a disease trigger affective reactions, perception of controllability and subsequent personal control-related activities, which people use to recover from the aversive consequences of a health problem. These conditions need to be incorporated in a theoretical model to make recovery sufficiently predictable.

Studies in this field have primarily focused on the kind of causal attributions people make for different health problems. It is just not enough to find the kind of causal explanations people have for their health problems. Understanding of the causal explanations that people give should form the basis to address questions related to other antecedents of their overall recovery. The questions, such as why do some people become angry and frustrated in the face of a health crisis while others just stoically accept their suffering? Why are some people more emotionally upset than others, and why others keep a positive profile? Why some are actively involved in the treatment procedure while others resign to their fate and feel helpless? When do people exercise control over their environment and when do they try to accommodate themselves according to the demands of the situation? When do people strongly react to the loss of control, when do they willingly give up control? How are the health-related attributions which people make embedded in their socio-economic background?

Obviously, one single research project or theoretical formulation cannot answer all these questions. No theory can be broad enough to account for all diversities in the way people respond to their health crises. In spite of all research in this domain, we are at the very initial stage of understanding the complexities of the human mind and its infinite capacity to reconstruct a situation and react differently. No psychological theory can encompass all these complexities, as each person responds to an illness situation in his or her unique ways.

However, in this chapter we endeavour to develop a comprehensive model to understand the interplay of those psychosocial factors that play a crucial role in the overall recovery of a person from the disease. Psychophysical recovery, as will be discussed in more detail in later chapters, does not have any fixed goals, nor can it be conceived as an end state, but is seen as an ongoing process with all ups and downs. Recovery from a chronic condition is a long-drawn process, often lifelong and goes through the vicissitudes of stages, with relapses and remissions, with setbacks and speedy recovery, which may drain psychosocial and financial resources of the diseased person and his/her family. Any model of such recovery, no matter how comprehensive it may be, cannot account for all patterns of responses. The attributional model of psychological recovery proposed in this chapter is tentative in this sense.

The proposed model has at the core beliefs which people have about the chronic disease, both, those which caused the problem and those which contribute to their recovery. Such disease-related attributions are the products of our own belief system, part of which we inherit during our enculturation and part of which we develop due to our life experiences. It may be contended that such beliefs, which are referred to as attributions are dynamic and context-specific. There is a wide variability in these attributional beliefs across people and different disease conditions, but also across different stages of the same disease for the same person. Such attributions serve some purpose for the attributor of which she may or may not be aware. Such self-service reflect in the way people judge the severity of their problems, take time in deciding about the remedial measures and show actual recovery. A more systematic understanding of the way in which causal beliefs lead to certain other cognitions and actions is essential and could account for some of the inconsistencies in the existing research.

The proposed attributional model can show up when patients of chronic diseases construe a positive appraisal of the situation to mobilize their internal resources. The model can map the consequences of various curative intervention strategies. It should make it possible to identify those causal and recovery attributions that facilitate and those which impede recovery. Many attributional change programmes have been developed in recent years to modify dysfunctional attributions. This model can facilitate development of attribution therapies, which can change dysfunctional attributions. The chronically ill treat themselves with the help of their doctor, family, friends and other people in their social network. Studies (Dweck, 1975; Forsterling, 1985) have demonstrated the efficacy of the attribution therapy in the treatment of various emotional disorders.

The proposed attributional model of psychological recovery is essentially a cognitive model, as the focus is on causal and recovery beliefs. Such beliefs are off-course, closely linked with affective and behavioural responses. Before we present this model, it may be a good exercise to familiarize ourselves with some existing cognitive approaches that have relevance to understand patient behaviour in a disease condition.

A Review of Some Cognitive Approaches

There are few theoretical approaches that have enhanced our understanding of the reactions to undesirable life events from the patients' perspective. The theoretical models presented here fall in the broad domain of cognitive approach based on patients' own construction of the event and its consequences. These models are often employed to understand the health behaviour of patients with chronic diseases. The formulation of the attributional theory of psychological recovery has been built over these theoretical approaches.

Lazarus Theory of Cognitive Appraisal

Though not dealing with causal appraisal, Lazarus (1966, 2000) has been the pioneer in investigating cognitive variables for their role in coping with stressful events. In an initial study, Lazarus and colleagues (1970) analysed reactions to stressful events in terms of cognitive processes that mediate encounters between the person and his environment that leads to adaptational outcomes. The theory deals with three types of appraisals, each of which serves in its own fashion to moderate the encounter. The first is primary appraisal, which is a cognitive process of evaluation of the significance of an encounter for one's well-being. This takes place immediately after the onset of the stressful event. This appraisal is in terms of the nature of the event, its severity and implications for one's life. The second is secondary appraisal, which is the process of evaluating an encounter with respect to coping resource and options. People assign causal meaning, assess their internal resources, comprehend the overall impact of the crisis on their life, the kind of adjustment they would be required to make, etc. These are the major considerations at this stage. The third is reappraisal, which occurs as new information is obtained from internal psychological changes, from changes in the environment because of coping efforts, from further assessment, and from defensive intrapsychic activity, which is also a kind of coping.

The conceptual system presented by Lazarus and his colleagues emphasized the role of cognition in shaping emotional reactions to tragic events. According to Lazarus (1966), one of the objectives of the coping strategy that a person in crisis uses is to reduce or regulate the emotional response itself, so as to minimize its detrimental effects. This is done by a variety of intrapsychic or cognitive coping processes, such as avoidance, intellectualized detachment and denial. If the person tries not to think about the harm or danger and succeeds, there will be no anxiety; if the danger is denied, again the distress is short circuited; and if the personal emotional implications of a tragedy are distanced or examined with detachment as an intellectual exercise, the potential emotional reactions are reduced by the cognitive regulating process. In fact, if the emotional reaction is intense, coping is first directed at regulating emotions. This may be done by reappraising the event as less threatening or less important.

The theory contends that the range of coping strategies, which can be simultaneously or sequentially employed, is very wide, encompassing at least four main categories: information search, direct action, inhibition of action and intrapsychic mode. These coping resources are not static in the sense that they depend on experience, degree of stress and adaptational requirements. Depending on the circumstances, the coping strategy employed has two main functions, namely to alter the person environment relationship (problem-solving) or to regulate stressful emotional reactions.

Brehm's Theory of Reactance

Reactance is a response of anger and hostility to loss of control when already existing or expected control is arbitrarily threatened or withdrawn. According to Brehm (1966; Brehm and Brehm, 1981), reactance in a given setting would depend upon the severity of threat, and importance of freedom for the patients. In this setting, if the behaviour is restricted, people react with a feeling of hostility, anger and enhanced motivation to obtain the outcome in question. Clearly, there is a contradiction between the helplessness model and reactance theory. Wortman and Behm (1975) revised the existing model to resolve this contradiction. This model predicts that among individuals who expect to be able to influence the outcome, exposure to loss of control results in enhanced motivation to obtain the outcome, and aggressive and angry behaviour. However, expectations of control should diminish overtime as people make repeated but unsuccessful attempts to change the situation. Once a person stops trying to change the situation, continued exposure to it should result in lowered motivation, passivity and depression. This integrative model has yet to be tested empirically.

Weiner's Attributional Theory of Motivation and Emotions

Though both the learned helplessness model and reactance theory have incorporated causal beliefs to explain affective reactions, a more comprehensive attributional theory is propounded by Weiner (1985). The theory assumes that causal search precedes all affective reactions. Taking lead from the work of Heider (1958) and Kelley (1967), Weiner suggested that all causal beliefs could be characterized by three dimensions of locus, stability and controllability. The locus of causality dimension refers to whether the attributed cause is internal to the person (personality traits, skills, efforts made, etc.) or external to him or her (chance, lack of facilities, pollution, etc.). The stability dimension also has two levels: stable or unstable causes; whether the attributed cause is going to persist over time or is just transitory. For example, efforts can vary over time (unstable cause), but personality trait may be stable over time. Similarly, attributed causes could be within the control of a person (efforts made, self-care, etc.) or uncontrollable (fate, etc.).

According to Weiner, different causal dimensions are associated with different psychological reactions. Attributing the event to internal factors is predicted to affect the self-esteem of the person. For example, if he or she thinks that illness is because of his/her own carelessness, it would lower his/her self-esteem. Attribution to external factors protects one's self-esteem. The stability dimension is related to future expectations. Attribution of recovery to stable factors would lead to higher expectations of recovery in future. The controllability dimension predicts how much effort people are going to make on their part, or would show a sense of helplessness.

The theory also posits that different emotions are associated with different causal dimensions. The self-esteem-related affective reactions (such as shame, feeling of incompetence, worthlessness) are dependent on attribution to internal factors. The expectation-related affective reactions (such as hope, disappointment and depression) are elicited by attribution to stable causes. The controllability dimension is associated with feelings of guilt, anger, helplessness, etc. It may, however, be stated that most of the work to test these propositions were conducted in the achievement domain. There are very few studies testing these linkages in the context of tragic life events.

Weiner's theory has been extensively examined in a wide range of situations—from examination performance to automobile accidents. Dalal and Sethi (1987) tested this theory in the Indian culture and found support for the cross-cultural generality of the theory.

Theory of Cognitive Adaptation

Taylor (1983) proposed a comprehensive theory of cognitive adaptation suggesting that people are motivated to have a positive subjective construction of their sickness. A positive cognitive appraisal is essential to have better adjustment in a stressful situation. One thing that people do is to make causal attributions in such a manner that they can retain some sense of personal control. They put the blame on those factors that are modifiable, such as carelessness, and can be controlled in future. Their hopes in a better future thus remain untampered. Secondly, patients, even those who are severely injured or ill, engage in positive comparison, thinking it could have been worse, or that they are much better off than others and are more fortunate. This conscious effort to make a positive comparison makes them feel good. Third aspect of the cognitive adaptation theory is that people tend to preserve a positive self-esteem by appraising the situation in such a way that they can absolve themselves of self-blame for the things going wrong. Taylor did a series of studies on cancer patients and general support for her theoretical formulation. The theory makes many interesting propositions, which deserve further empirical support.

Theories of Learned Helplessness and Learned Optimism

The theory of learned helplessness (Seligman, 1975) was originally proposed to account for laboratory data on reactions to uncontrollable outcomes. Learned helplessness occurs, when an individual concludes from repeated failure that the termination of an aversive outcome is independent of his/her responses. In essence, the theory predicts that in the face of repeated encounter with tragic events the individual may give in and stop making efforts. This realization that one's responses do not alter the uncontrollable state generalizes to other events where control is actually possible. These people thus develop depressive tendencies and show performance deficit. The theory was in the first place tested on animals.

In the later reformulation of the theory (Abramson et al., 1978), it was contended that the kind of causal attributions people make for lack of control will affect their self-esteem and the degree to which their symptoms of helplessness and depression will generalize across situations and time. The theory, however, does not predict other emotional reactions. So far the support for this theory has come from experimental work where controllable situations are much simplified and where few response alternatives are available. Though the theory has many implications for examining reactions to chronic illnesses, such researches are not evident. The cross-cultural research that has been conducted suggests that while learned helplessness is similarly manifested in other cultures of Europe, Storey (2008) has found evidence that bicultural Native Americans experienced less frustration in a learned helplessness situation than traditional Native Americans.

Seligman (1998) further reformulated his theoretical proposition of helplessness to incorporate optimism as an alternative explanatory style in the same crisis situation. Rather than taking a negative view, a person in that situation may arrive at an optimistic explanation by changing his/her casual attributions. Thus, a person may learn to be optimistic by making external (external situation, other person), unstable (negative outcome is not likely to reoccur) and specific attribution (only in case of this event). Such causal attribution for negative events creates a mental state of learned optimism. Such learned optimism is likely to result in better physical health and more effective coping strategies in an adverse situation (Peterson, 2000).

Theory of Learned Resourcefulness and Resilience

Rosenbaum (1990) developed a theory of learned resourcefulness that suggested that individuals who are resourceful cope better with stress than those who are poor in resourcefulness. Learned resourcefulness is an acquired repertoire of self-control skills by which a person self-regulates internal states (both negative and positive) for the smooth execution of a desired behaviour. According to the theory, these self-control skills are important for attaining, maintaining or regaining health in the face of adverse situations. People high on resourcefulness are better able to deal with crises situations in a more adaptive, constructive manner than persons with low resourcefulness. Resourceful people have better quality of life and have better adaptation in the face of life adversities. They are more effective in dealing with emotions and demanding situation. Research has shown that patients who are resourceful and self-efficacious have more positive self-appraisals and were likely to receive more social support. Such people are better able to manage their chronic illnesses by mobilizing requisite resources to deal with debilitating illness episodes (Frydenberg, 2004).

A related concept is psychological resilience, which refers to the individual's ability to withstand the challenge of life and life stresses (Weiss, 2008). Resilience is the positive side of vulnerability. It refers to one's ability to bounce back from adversity; it does not mean that one will not be wounded, but would emerge from it as a stronger person (Werner and Smith, 1992). Resilient people have positive appraisal of the situation, high on morality (spirituality), cognitively flexible and have positive self-concept. These characteristics put resilience in the same category of concepts as the learned resourcefulness is. However, whereas learned resourcefulness is an acquired repertoire of strategies and skills (mostly cognitive), resilience is both acquired and inborn, they serve the same objectives for the person (Dalal, 2012). Furthermore, resilience is taken as developmental–dispositional characteristic; children acquire resilience in the developmental process to deal with life challenges. Resilience is commonly understood both as a process and a disposition.

Commonsense Model of Illness Perception

In the *common sense model* patients' perception of their illness and threat to health are key concepts, which trigger the self-regulation process (Leventhal et al., 1984). According to this model, people make sense of a health threat by developing their own cognitive and emotional representations of that threat. These representations or perceptions develop from exposure to a variety of social and cultural sources of information—news stories, education in schools, personal experiences of illness, witnessing illness experiences of others, portrayals of illness in books and movies, and other experiences (Cameron and Caza, 2004). Common sense model postulates that both cognitive and emotional representations determine how patients cope and adapt to their illness. The representations generally consist of the following components:

- *identity*—patients' beliefs about the label of the illness and associated symptoms;
- *cause*—patients' beliefs about factors or conditions that have caused the illness;
- *timeline*—patients' beliefs about the expected duration of the illness;
- *personal control*—patients' beliefs about how much their own actions will help to control the illness;
- *treatment control*—patients' beliefs about how much their prescribed treatment will be effective in controlling or curing the condition;
- *consequences*—patients' beliefs about the impact of the illness on their physical, social and psychological well-being;
- *coherence*—patients' beliefs about how well they understand the illness;
- *representation of emotional reaction*—patients' beliefs about how much they are emotionally affected by the illness, for example, whether they experience fear or worry.

All these beliefs taken together determine the course of action which a patient will take.

Bandura's Self-efficacy Theory

Self-efficacy is a psychological mechanism that has been shown to mediate physiologic outcomes and health-related behaviour (Bandura, 1977, 1997). Perceived self-efficacy represents an individual's perception of how capable he or she is of performing a specific activity or task, predicts whether a specific activity will be attempted, and determines how long the individual will persevere in the face of significant challenges. Perceived self-efficacy also relates to an individual's process of deciding what response he or she will make, how much effort will be put forth, and how much stress will be experienced. The self-efficacy predicts whether a specific activity will be attempted or a recommended regimen of exercise and diet will be adhered to or not (Gardner et al., 2003). Gardner and colleagues found that when self-efficacy was statistically controlled, the relationships among the other factors dramatically reduced.

The concept of self-efficacy was further extended at a collective level involving family, friends and communities. Collective self-efficacy is defined as 'the extent to which we believe that we can work together effectively to accomplish our shared goals' (Maddux, 2009, p. 340). This premise is not fully developed, not tested empirically but seems to have the potential to examine how our beliefs in the effectiveness of significant others contribute to psychological recovery of chronic patients.

A feature common to all these theoretical models presented above is that they are cognitive in orientation. Their real-life applications are limited by the inherent shortcomings of human information processing system, errors and biases that influence human judgments. Any action would depend on how particular information is processed, elaborated or discounted. This is a dynamic process that changes not only from one chronic condition to the other but also in the same disease condition when the context changes (Crano and Prislin, 2006; Fazio and Olson, 2002). Furthermore, people use multiple cognitive strategies available or invented, and choose among them depending on the goals, intentions and resources available. Often people use heuristic rules, such as 'doctors know the best', 'destiny is powerful' and 'patient needs support', which influence decision-making and actions in a chronic condition (Kruglanski and Orehek, 2007). Cultural beliefs, thus, become potent considerations in dealing with chronic health crisis. One such culturally constructed formulation is the doctrine of Karma, which is subscribed by the overwhelming majority of Hindus and others.

The Hindu Doctrine of Karma

The Hindu doctrine of Karma is a cultural belief model that is subscribed to explain many serious health crises. The doctrine of Karma as stated in Indian scriptures since olden times shapes behaviour in many life domains, including health. This doctrine has evolved over thousands of years and there are several variations in its formulation. Here, we restrict our discussion to only those tenets that are relevant in the context of psychological recovery. It states that the balance of good and bad deeds accumulates over all previous lives and if someone has done bad deeds in previous births he may have to suffer for the same in this life (Paranjpe, 1984). This principle not only restores one's faith in a just world but also provides a very convincing and socially acceptable explanation for a host of undesirable events.

The other tenet relevant in the present context is that one should strive to attain a state of detachment, in which the outcome of the event, whatever it may be, does not cause emotional crisis for the person. According to the Gita, one can attain this state by systematically training oneself for mental equipoise. Once this state is achieved, the person neither desires nor feels sad, whatever the outcome may be. According to Radhakrishna (1926), this doctrine of Karma is so deep-rooted in the Hindu psyche that most of the tragic events are interpreted from this perspective. Very frequently, its tenets are invoked to facilitate the recovery process. Though not much empirical evidence is available, in a study conducted by Pande and Naidu (1986) it was found that task orientation (detachment) reduces strain in a stressful situation.

It was observed in a number of studies that the theory of Karma is often invoked by the patients and their families to understand and explain a wide range of social and personal happenings. Such attributions have implications for psychological recovery of the suffering of individuals and their families. This phenomenon will be evident in the studies reported in this volume and will be discussed over and again.

As stated earlier, these cognitive orientations discussed above primarily focus on how people structure their experiences in a crisis situation, learn from their experiences and make necessary changes in their cognitions so as to evolve effective strategies to combat the crisis. However, these theories have two general limitations. Firstly, though these theories attempt to predict reactions to chronic diseases, they are not primarily concerned with how people who recover employ these diseases. It is not clear what strategies people form to regain a sense of personal control and what role this sense of personal control has in recovering from the disease. Secondly, these theories do not underlie the sequence through which cognitions translate into certain remedial action tendencies. The ways people causally appraise the situation have many implications for their subsequent responses but these are not clearly brought out in these theories. Building on these existing theoretical formulations, this chapter proposes a theory of psychological recovery in which causal beliefs are of central importance.

Why Me? The Causal Search

'Why has this disease happened to me, not to anyone else?' is a question that often haunts the suffering individuals. People often need an answer to reconcile with a major health crisis. There is enough research evidence to suggest that people spontaneously engage in causal search to have a rather convincing explanation. In a review of 26 published research studies, Weiner (1985) found strong evidence for causal thinking. However, this causal thinking does not trigger on every conceivable occasion. Wong and Weiner (1981) and Weiner (1985) found that causal search is activated when the outcome is negative and unexpected. In an experimental study taking a student sample, Dalal and Agrawal (1987) confirmed that negative outcome promotes causal search. The motivation to find causes of the illness was recognized in many early clinical studies of cancer patients (e.g. Bard and Dyk, 1956). Patients were found to be reporting perceived cause of their illness, when questioned about it, following their diagnosis. In the research that assessed patients months and years after the diagnosis, the number of patients who reported causal attributions ranged from 69% to 95% (Affleck et al., 1985). In another study, Taylor et al. (1984) found that a majority of cancer patients, their spouses, relatives and close friends do report the causes of cancer. However, the frequency of causal attributions varies with the type of illness. Lung cancer patients were less likely to report causes of their illness than myocardial infarction patients (Mumma and McCorkle, 1982). Frequency of the attributed causes also depends on the severity of illness. Cardiac patients with more severe symptoms reported more causal attributions than those who had less severe symptoms (Affleck et al., 1985). It was shown by French et al. (2010) that in case of first myocardial infarction patient, their causal attributions may be realistic, but not predictive of subsequent changes in behaviour.

Studies conducted on Indian hospitalized patients present a somewhat different picture. Two studies, by Dalal and Pande (1988) and Dalal and Singh (1992) on orthopaedic and tuberculosis patients, respectively, addressed this issue. The results showed that causal thinking was not very frequent among orthopaedic patients with accidental injuries. The patients were asked whether they contemplated why this mishap occurred to only them. Most of the answers fell in the categories 'never' (1) and 'seldom' (2) on a 5-point scale. When the patients were specifically asked to mention the causes of the accident, most of them gave one or two causes; permanently disabled listing less causes than the temporarily disabled. In the second study on tuberculosis patients, it was found that very few patients mentioned more than one cause. In another study by Agrawal and Dalal (1993) on heart attack patients, a similar pattern was observed.

Most of the studies to date have typically examined causal explanations in terms of types of causal attributions made in relation to health and illness. Such research has primarily relied on the three-dimensional analysis of causal attributions, as internal–external, stable–unstable and controllable–uncontrollable, following Weiner's classification (Weiner, 1985). Any chronic disease is a complex situation and likely to involve complex attributions that are often interdependent (Sensky, 1997). Such illness beliefs are integral to the larger belief system, which a person subscribes to. Further, such causal beliefs about the illness are perceived within the temporarily ordered network of interconnected causes and effects. Such perceived cause–effect linkages acquire different meanings in different cultures (Vaughn et al., 2009).

It is, however, argued that low evidence for causal thinking does not necessarily imply absence of causal beliefs. A number of causal beliefs are part of the cultural belief system, deeply ingrained in the process of socialization. In all the three studies referred above, God's will and Karma were more frequently mentioned as causes by the Hindu patients implying greater acceptance of their fate, rather than questioning it. This finding is corroborated in other studies too (e.g. Priya, 2010).

Whether causal search is present or absent, the evidence is overwhelming that the patients who have causal explanations are better adjusted than those who have no causal explanations (Bulman and Wortman, 1977; Dalal and Singh, 1996; Silver and Wortman, 1980). Why do people need to have causes for their misfortune and suffering? There are several tentative answers. People generally do not want to believe that the world around them is chaotic and unlawful where events occur randomly. They need to find some order and meaning in the things happening to them and others. Frankl (1963) in a study of people who survived in the concentration camps during the Second World War found that this search for meaning in life was a major preoccupation of the prisoners. Those prisoners who could find a positive meaning in their suffering did cope better than the others. Paranjpe (1984, 1987) noted that the search for explanations of suffering has been the cornerstone of Indian philosophical traditions. By understanding the causes of an event, one may also begin to understand the significance of the event and what it symbolizes about one's life (Taylor, 1983). This understanding helps one to adjust to the new realities of life.

The other function that causal attributions serve for a patient is of assigning moral responsibility for the events. People generally want to believe in a just world (Lerner, 1975), where they get what they deserve and deserve what they get. It was observed by Lerner and his colleagues in a series of experiments (Lerner, 1975; Lerner and Matthews, 1967) that people have a tendency to blame the victims for their misfortunes. Bulman and Wortman (1977) found that the spinal cord injury patients who blamed themselves for the accident showed better coping than those who blamed others. Surprisingly, patients who coped better also believed that the accident was unavoidable. Bulman and Wortman explained this unusual finding in terms of the fact that the patients believed that they were voluntarily engaged in the activity that led to the accident. The motivation to make attribution appears much more complex in view of the finding that those accident victims who attributed their accident to Karma showed better recovery (Dalal and Pande, 1988), whereas, in the case of tuberculosis patients this finding was not supported (Dalal and Singh, 1992). More work is required to understand the implications of the belief in Karma. Western studies have completely ignored such beliefs.

Attribution to Karma implies blaming oneself in causal but not in moral terms. In a few studies, the distinction between causal and moral responsibility is maintained. It is quite possible to blame oneself in a causal sense but not in the moral sense (Kanekar, 1988). For example, when you ignore normal health precautions, violate normal procedures or take unnecessary risk, you may believe yourself to be causally responsible but not morally. The essence of this aspect of explanation is the question of what you ought to have done, rather than the consequences of what you did. In a study of accident victims by Brewin (1984), greater causal self-blame was associated with victims feeling less anxious and tense, whereas greater moral self-blame was associated with early return to work.

Quite often, making attributional judgments is a public activity and people are supposed to communicate why they fell sick. People generally want to present themselves favourably in the eyes of others and make esteem-enhancing, self-protective attributions. Snyder et al. (1976) refer to this tendency as egotism and suggest that when faced with the possibility of failure on a task, people may apply the tactics of not trying or of giving up prematurely. This has the advantage that people can attribute their failure to lack of effort, a less distressing cause than lack of ability. Hirt and others (2003) found the evidence of people using various self-handicapping strategies to have some face-saving causal attributions.

Recovery Beliefs

It is surprising that causal beliefs were so extensively investigated but recovery beliefs were hardly paid any attention to by the researchers in this area. Research shows that patients are not only keen to understand the causes of their illness but are equally eager to figure out the factors that will contribute to their recovery. Recovery beliefs imply the factors to which patients attribute their physical recovery and the presence of these factors is considered necessary for further recovery from the disease or its harmful effects. In fact, our research has shown that in some cases, recovery beliefs are better predictors of recovery than the causal beliefs.

Causal and recovery beliefs differ in many ways. Whereas causal beliefs are based on some retrospective analysis of the occurrence of disease, reconstructing the event and inferring causality; recovery beliefs are prospective in nature, the analysis of the contributing factors is based on the goals of the treatment or the state of health people want to retain. Secondly, the inference of causality has an implication for prediction or prevention of the recurrence of the disease or its acute stage, inference about the recovery factors is essential to direct the efforts and predict recovery. Thirdly, temporally recovery beliefs are closer to recovery than causal beliefs. Though the contents of the causal and recovery beliefs could be the same, for example, God's will could be both a causal and recovery belief, but its psychological meaning would differ. God's will as a cause would imply punishment from God, but as a recovery belief it would mean his benevolence. Scanning of literature shows that Brickman and his associates made a similar distinction in the study of helping behaviour-incorporating causal attribution and personal control in a unifying model. Brickman and others (1982) made a distinction between attribution of responsibility for the problem and for its solution. Four alternative situations were examined, giving rise to four different models. People may hold themselves responsible for both the cause and the solution (moral model); for causing the disease only but not for the solution (enlightenment model); not for causing the problem but for its solution (compensatory model), neither for causing nor for the solution of the problem (hospital model). Helping behaviour was found to be varying in these four situations.

Though this model was initially proposed to predict helping behaviour but it can be applied in cases of chronic illness (Dalal, 1988, 1999). Our earlier studies (Dalal, 2000) have shown that causal and recovery beliefs have both emotional and behavioural implications and affect recovery of the patients. On the basis of our own and others' researches in the related areas, we have formulated our cognitive (attributional) model of psychological recovery as a part of broader psychomedical model.

Proposed Cognitive (Attributional) Model of Psychological Recovery

The proposed model (Figure 3.1) views chronic disease from the perspective of the person suffering from a chronic disease. As stated earlier, the context of a chronic disease is different from that of acute and terminal diseases, where recovery is mostly at home and long-range planning is required to deal with the crisis. In case of chronic disease, a person gets sufficient time to examine various causal propositions before arriving at relatively stable attributions. Members of the family and close social network often join in such a review process.

Some basic assumptions about human nature are implicit in this proposed model. First, it views people capable of self-healing, as having energy not only for withstanding setbacks, but also for attaining a higher level of efficiency. Two, the model assumes that in most of the

Figure 3.1:
Schematic outline of the proposed attributional model of psychological recovery

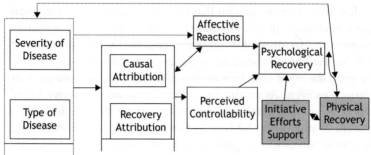

cases people do not seek external (or institutional) help to face the crisis; they rather generate their own inner resources to deal with it. People in crisis quite frequently exhibit learned resourcefulness. Three, people, in general, are motivated to appraise the event, look for the best alternatives, have some kind of feedback system and are the best informers about their own illness.

Furthermore, the proposed attributional model of psychological recovery assumes the centrality of causal and recovery attributions in recovering from a long-term illness or disability. These attributional inferences about the disease and recovery sets in an internal response chain leading to a subjective construction of the health problem and coming up with the response strategies, which are appropriate to the demands of the situation. The model assumes that perception of causality and recovery factors may change depending on appraisal and reappraisal of the situation in which members of family and social network joins.

More specifically, the proposed model posits that the causal attributions and perception of control are interdependent. Perceived causes that are held responsible for the chronic illness provide the basis for categorizing the event as personally controllable, personally uncontrollable, controllable by others or universally uncontrollable. It is equally likely that if the individual has strong preconceptions about the controllability of life events in general, these will guide the search for those causes, which are personally controllable. Our cultural beliefs provide a larger framework within which search for the causes of a specific disease takes place. Also, an unexpected or novel event may justify the primacy of causal search. In either case, perceived causality provides the basis for considering whether a particular event is controllable or not.

It is important to mention that the endeavour is not just to understand how people make attribution for both—the causes of the chronic problem and factors people consider responsible for their own recovery, but also their possible affective, evaluative and action-related outcomes. In brief, the effort is to link attributions with their psychological and physical recovery. As we all know, predicting recovery is a very hazardous venture and research findings in this area are still very tentative. A chronic disease is stressful on a long-term basis, where the debilitating condition of the disease goes through different stages, and with that the emotions and perceptions of the suffering individual also fluctuate. People use different coping strategies in case of chronic diseases to figure out what works. It often renders psychological recovery as a transitory state, not a stable state of being.

The proposed model has been built on our empirical research and on other related theoretical and empirical work in this area. Attribution is a cognitive process, that is, a conscious process, and it can account for only those affective states and thinking, which are rational and deliberate. Since in the case of chronic diseases, much of the coping is in terms of integrating the disease in the life, a good deal of decision-making and adjustments are towards achieving that goal. One has to think, plan, consult and seek cooperation of family and social network to deal with the ongoing crisis. This cognitive processing should enable this model to predict to a larger extent, psychological recovery.

According to the proposed model, whenever people encounter a chronic disease, their initial effort is to grasp its perceived severity, in terms of potentially adverse consequences of the problem. It seems logical to conjecture that perceived severity will be inversely associated with psychological recovery. This cognitive appraisal of the disease and the nature of problem will trigger the causal search process, in which case, the patient actively seeks out the causes of his/her illness. Previous researches (Dalal and Weiner, 1988; Wong and Weiner, 1981) have shown that this search will be intense when the outcome is undesirable or unexpected. Patients not only seek causes of the problem, but also appraise what will contribute to their recovery from it. This attributional process may continue over a long period, and people may arrive at different combinations of perceived causes at different stages of the disease and recovery.

Such causal and recovery attributions provide the basis to patients/ people to further appraise controllability of the disease. There could be four ways of appraising controllability of an event. As mentioned earlier, these are—personally controllable, personally uncontrollable, controllable by others and universally uncontrollable. Personal and cultural beliefs play a major role in the attribution of the disease, as well as, in appraisal of its controllability. Furthermore, causal and recovery attributions, and perceived severity of the disease should determine affective responses of the person/patient. It is contended though that some generalized affective reactions are dependent on the severity of the disease *per se*. There are other affective reactions, such as anger, depression, hopelessness, fear, guilt and contempt, which are attribution-dependent.

Perceived controllability and affective reactions in combination will determine psychological recovery of the person/patient. There are many other factors, such as personal initiative and efforts of the patient, family and health professionals, including the support of social network, which are crucial in psychological and physical recovery. However, these are not part of the cognitive (attributional) model of psychological recovery. The proposed model is primarily concerned with cognitive antecedents of psychological recovery. It may, however, be mentioned that no direct linkages were found between psychological and physical recovery in the literature. This linkage is mediated by many other considerations. This is the reason why these two sets of variables are shaded in the proposed model.

UNIT II

Beliefs about Chronic Diseases

4

Psychological Recovery of Accident Victims with Physical Disability*

A great deal of research has accumulated in the last two decades to predict psychological recovery of the victims of tragic events. Much of this work has focussed on affective reactions (Shontz, 1975; Weller and Miller, 1976; Wortman and Brehm, 1975), coping strategies (Goldiamon, 1975; Lazarus, 1966), behavioral consequences like learned helplessness (Abramson et al., 1978; Miller and Norman, 1979), and causal beliefs (Bulman and Wortman, 1977; Shaver, 1970; Thompson, 1981). Taken as a whole, these studies reveal lack of consensus about the predictors of reactions to tragic events (see Silver and Wortman, 1980). Expressing similar views, Taylor has stated, 'though many systematic attempts are made, our knowledge of those factors that influence our reactions to tragic outcomes is very vague' (1983: 1161).

It may further be mentioned that the role of beliefs about self, causality and personal control in the recovery process have not been sufficiently understood. Many of these beliefs have their anchoring in

* Reproduced from Dalal, A.K. and Pande, N. (1988). Psychological recovery of the accident victims with temporary and permanent disability. In Dalal, A.K. and Misra, G. (2002). *New Directions in Indian Psychology: Social Psychology*, vol. 1. New Delhi: SAGE Publications.

Namita Pande is Professor of Psychology at the University of Allahabad, Allahabad. This text has been edited for typographical errors, stylistic consistency, and sequential organization in order to make it suitable for inclusion in this book.

specific socio-cultural context. For example, the principle of Karma, as expounded in Hinduism, is widely accepted as an explanation for many tragic happenings in one's life. The goal of the present study thus was to examine how these beliefs influence psychological recovery of temporarily and permanently disabled accident victims.

How do people react to tragic accidents? The initial reaction may be that of shock and confusion. At the early stage, the impinging reality may seem too overwhelming to allow any luxury of cognitive appraisal of the whole situation. However, subsequent reactions of the victims would depend on the way the causality for that event is attributed. The understanding of these causes gives a sense of personal control over their environment, without which the world would seem random and chaotic. Studies have shown that those who have rather convincing answers to the question, 'why it has happened to me?' are psychologically better off than those who have no such explanations available (Bulman and Wortman, 1977; Weisman and Worden, 1975).

The attribution of causality to the event would determine whether the victim would feel angry, or feel helpless. The victim would experience anger when the cause of the accident is attributed to factors controllable by others (e.g. carelessness, rash driving). According to Abramson et al. (1978), learned helplessness occurs when people perceive the event uncontrollable and attribute it to stable-internal causes (e.g. poor eyesight, nervousness). These people would be depressed, and would show withdrawal symptoms. Rosenbaum and Ben-Ari (1985) demonstrated that in many instances, instead of learned helplessness, people show learned resourcefulness to effectively cope with the crisis.

Reviewing a large number of studies, Rothbaum et al. (1982) suggested that withdrawal symptoms, characteristic of learned helplessness, may in fact be an attempt to change one's own cognitions so as to 'bring own-self into line with the environmental forces'. Learned resourcefulness depends on the ability and willingness to use self-control skills in order to reduce the interfering effects of emotions and cognitions. People high on learned resourcefulness were expected to experience less distress and focus more on the recovery.

This type of self-directed behavior, according to Rothbaum (1983), is motivated to gain secondary control, when efforts to have primary control (changing the aversive conditions itself) fall. For example, attributing the accident to one's own poor eyesight can serve to enhance predictive secondary control and protect oneself against future distress;

attribution to powerful others (e.g. God) permits vicarious secondary control when the individual identifies him/herself with them. Thus if people, particularly people in crises, will strive to change external conditions if they can, otherwise they will resort to secondary control.

People not only make efforts to gain some amount of control, but at times are actively involved in seeking meaning in their sufferings (Frankl, 1963). In the face of a tragic event, many people desire to maintain their faith in a just world. According to the just world hypothesis (Lerner, 1971), people tend to belief that one gets what one deserves and that misdeeds are always punished. In many cultures, faith in just world is deep-rooted and transmitted through socialization process. The tragic accidents may shake this faith causing additional stress. To restore faith in a just world people view their suffering as a punishment from God, something they deserved for their misdeeds. Such people tend to blame themselves for the accident. In Hindu culture particularly, belief in the principle of Karma implies that good and bad deeds accumulate over all previous lives and if someone is suffering, he or she must have done some wrong in the previous lives. As interpreted by Paranjpe (1984), the principle of Karma is based on determinism that all human behavior is lawful and no one can escape experiences of joy or suffering as the consequences of his own past deeds. This principle not only restores one's faith in justice but also provides a very convincing and socially acceptable explanation for the event. There is not enough empirical evidence to this date to predict influence of faith in Karma on recovery of the accident victims.

A review of the literature reveals that the term psychological recovery is treated as a multifaceted concept. The indicators of successful recovery included in various studies are keeping one's distress within manageable limits, having a positive self-concept, hopefulness, positive and realistic view of the situation and clarity of future plans (e.g. Haan, 1977; Hamburg and Adams, 1967). However, many studies have cast doubts on the validity of some of these indices. For example, Goldsmith (1955) reported patients with spinal cord injuries, who were more distressed about their disability and expressed anger and aggressive feeling about what happened to them, were subsequently judged as showing more progress in rehabilitation than those who appeared less distressed. Similar findings were obtained in some other studies as well (e.g. Derogatis, 1977). It thus seems unwarranted at this stage to rely on only one measure of psychological recovery. The indicators in the present study included hopefulness, being active, clarity of future plans, efforts made and positive attitude. An overall index of recovery was also obtained.

The subject population of the present study consisted of accident victims who were getting treatment in a government hospital or in various nursing homes in Allahabad city. The patients were categorized as temporarily or permanently disabled from the accident. This population was selected for three reasons. First, the accident by nature catches a person unaware and there is no possibility of prior mental preparation, as in the case of a chronic disease. Hence, it is possible, in the case of an accident, to monitor the onset and nature of the coping process. Second, most of the orthopaedic patients need a prolonged treatment. Thus, data could be obtained under uniform conditions at different points in time. The drop-out rate is also minimal in such cases. Third, many studies have shown that psychological recovery will follow a different course for permanently disabled than for temporarily disabled patients (Bulman and Wortman, 1977; Thompson, 1982; Walster, 1966). Walster hypothesized that when the consequences of an accident become increasingly severe, people are more motivated to assign responsibility for the accident. The findings of Bulman and Wortman (1977) suggest that feeling of personal control (self-blame) may be adaptive when the outcome is modifiable, but can be maladaptive when the outcome is not modifiable, as in the case of permanently disabled patients. The present study aimed at testing these hypotheses on temporarily and permanently disabled patients.

Method

Sample

Forty-one patients receiving orthopaedic treatment at the Swaroop Rani Nehru Hospital and at other private nursing homes in Allahabad city, India, were studied. Patients who had received major injuries due to an accident in the previous week were selected on the basis of the doctor's report. Of these, 21 patients were rendered permanently disabled because of the accident (like amputation), whereas 20 patients, though badly injured, had chances of full recovery.

The age of these patients varied from 16 to 42 years. All of them except 3 were males, from both rural and urban background, mostly belonging to lower-middle-class Hindu families. Subsequent inquiry revealed that the overwhelming number of accidents was accounted for by road mishaps (48%). Fall from height, quarrel within family or neighborhood, trapped in transfer or oil machine were the causes of 14.6%, 14.1% and 14.6% of the cases, respectively. Anti-social elements, epileptic seizure, and saving someone from drowning were other instances of casualty. The nature of accidents for temporarily and permanently disabled patients showed similar patterns. Most of the patients got injuries (fracture) in the limbs. Patients in the first group had multiple injuries in 15% of the cases in comparison to 67% in the permanently disabled group.

Questionnaire

A questionnaire in Hindi was prepared. The initial items were related to the accident itself: circumstances of the accident, nature of injury sustained and progress of treatment. The next set of questions was about casual attributions. The opening item was an open-ended one about the factors responsible for the accident. The follow-up questions pertained to specific causes of the accident which were to be rated on a 5-point responsibility scale. Information about distress experienced and positive orientation was also sought. The psychological recovery was measured through the items related to perceived controllability, own efforts, future expectations, and attitude towards treatment. At the end, some demographic information was sought. The questionnaire was modified in the light of data obtained on a small sample.

Another questionnaire containing 10 items was also prepared to get the doctor's assessment of the patient's health. In particular, questions about the nature of injury, course of treatment, chances of recovery, and about mental health of the patient were included. These items were on a 5-point rating scale.

Data Collection

The patients were contacted individually with their doctor's permission while they were receiving treatment, or were waiting to be called in by the doctor. Since many of these patients were still in the state of shock and pain, it was apprehended that they may not like to talk. Contrary to this apprehension, the patients were quite willing to talk about the accident and liked to share their experience. As many of the patients were illiterate, care was taken to ensure that they had understood the questions. The administration of the questionnaire took about 30 to 40 minutes.

The attending doctor was also approached with a request to complete a small questionnaire for each of his patients participating in the study. He gave his assessment of the state of physical as well as psychological recovery of the patients.

The patients were approached again after approximately 15 days. The same questionnaire was administered and the doctor's report was again taken. There was no dropout.

Results

Psychological Stress Experienced

Some of the items in the questionnaire were indicative of the amount of stress experienced by the patients. Table 4.1 presents mean responses of temporary and permanent disability groups, 1 and 3 weeks after the accident. Separate 2 × 2, nature of injury × time, analyses of variance were computed, with time as a within-subject factor.

The first three items in Table 4.1 directly map the stress experienced by the patients. Though two groups of patients did not differ on these measures, the interaction on the item 'inconvenience experienced' was significant. This interaction revealed that at Time 1, both permanent and temporary disability groups exhibited same level of inconvenience (M = 4.50 and 4.65), but at Time 2, there was a marked difference in the inconvenience experienced (M = 4.60 and 3.30) by the two groups. As the time passed, temporarily disabled patients experienced less inconvenience. The findings were the same for the feeling of depression.

Items 4 and 5 (see Table 4.1) provided data on patients' rating of present crisis in comparison to the worst possible tragedy in one's life and the maximum possible injury in the same accident, respectively. Clearly, the permanently disabled person considered the accident more

Table 4.1:

Psychological stress experienced by patients with temporary and permanent disability at two time points

Questionnaire Item	Disability			Time Point			Interaction
	Permanent	*Temporary*	*F*	*1*	*2*	*F*	*F*
How much inconvenience are you experiencing?	4.55	3.98	3.90	4.58	3.95	8.68[b]	11.69[a]
How much anxiety do you have?	4.48	3.93	1.97	4.30	4.10	1.06	3.24
How much depression are you experiencing?	3.78	3.55	0.27	3.95	3.38	5.21[a]	2.84
Keeping in view the most tragic thing that can happen to you, how tragic is this accident?	4.64	3.78	4.82[a]	4.14	4.23	1.21	5.82
Keeping in view the injury you would have suffered due to this accident, how serious is the injury?	4.00	3.38	4.31[a]	3.84	4.04	0.86	3.41

[a] $p < 0.05$; [b] $p < 0.01$.

tragic than the temporarily disabled. The interaction effect on Item 4 further reveals that at Time 1, the mean difference between permanently and temporarily disabled was not marked ($M = 4.33$ and 3.95), but was so at Time 2 ($M = 4.95$ and 3.50). This implies that as the time passed, the accident was considered, more by the permanently than by the temporarily disabled group of patients, as a tragic happening in their lives. The pattern of mean ratings on Item 5 was also the same, though the interaction effect was statistically non-significant.

Causal Beliefs

To find the prevalence of causal content in the description of the event, content analysis was done by the two authors independently. The authors were kept incognizant of the patient's disability by mixing all descriptions. The description of the event as given by the patients was rated on 4-point scale (0 not present, 3 very much present). It was found that permanently disabled patients were significantly lower ($M = 1.28$) than the temporarily disabled ($M = 1.89$) on causal content. No other difference was significant.

The next item was 'do you contemplate why this has happened only to you?' The purpose was to check for the presence of egoistic causal thinking. The response range was from never (0) to always (5), with $M = 1.49$. None of the F ratios was significant in 2×2 analysis of variance. This mean rating is quite low (between never and seldom) implying that the 'why me only' question is not important from the patient's point of view.

The patients were then asked to state the possible causes of the accident. Most of the subjects gave one or two causes which again indicated a low prevalence of causal search. In fact, many of the patients stated that the accident was not caused—it just occurred. The causes stated by the subjects were categorized as internal, external or not clear, by three raters who were doctoral students in psychology. The frequencies of these causes are shown in Table 4.2.

Table 4.2 reveals different patterns of causal attributions for the two groups of patients. Permanently disabled patients attributed the accident more frequently to external than to internal factors. The pattern for temporarily disabled patients was different, as they equally attributed the causality to internal and external factors. This pattern of causality (not tested statistically as the frequencies were not independent) appears to be the same at two time points.

The patients then rated six specific causes assigning responsibility for the event. A 2×2 analysis of variance was computed for each causal category. Surprisingly none of the F ratios was significant. This implies that attributions of responsibility to the specific causes were not affected

Table 4.2:
Frequency of internal and external causes

Condition	*Internal*	*External*	*Unclear*	*No Cause*
Permanent disability				
Time 1	3	8	–	5
Time 2	2	6	1	7
Temporary disability				
Time 1	6	4	3	3
Time 2	4	5	4	1

by the nature of injury, nor did they change over time. The mean attributions on a 5-point scale for the six causal categories, Karma, own carelessness, others' carelessness, situation, chance and God's wishes were, respectively, 2.87, 2.59, 2.70, 1.68, 4.28 and 4.42. Clearly, higher attributions were made to chance and God's wishes.

Two other items measured perceived controllability on a 5-point scale. The patients in both conditions consistently stated that it was not possible to avoid the accident ($M = 1.64$). However, they reported that it would be possible for them to avoid such accidents in future ($M = 3.85$). This pattern was the same for the two groups across two time points.

The patients checked one of the seven factors as the most essential for recovery. There was a high degree of consistency in the factors listed by the patients on two occasions. More than half of the patients in both the groups gave God's will as the most important factor. Other factors considered as important facilitators of recovery by temporarily and permanently disabled patients were will power (22% and 7%) and proper treatment (17% and 22%). The temporarily disabled seems to have relied more on internal resources, whereas proper treatment was considered equally important by both groups.

Indices of Psychological Recovery

Some of the items in the questionnaire were taken to map psychological recovery. All these items were on a 5-point scale. The same 2 × 2 analyses of variance were computed for each of these items separately, as well as on the composite score of recovery. These results are summarized in Table 4.3.

It appears that hope of recovery (Item 1) was higher in the case of temporary disability than in the permanent one. Also, this hope of recovery augmented with time. On the other, four indices of recovery the differences between the two groups of patients were not significant, except in the case of clarity of future plans. The significant interaction in this case revealed that there was more clarity of future plans at Time 2 in the case of permanently disabled ($M = 1.97, 2.43$) as compared to temporarily disabled patients ($M = 2.58, 2.80$). The overall recovery score showed that recovery at Time 2 was better than at Time 1, which

Table 4.3:
2 × 2 Analysis of variance on the cognitive indices of psychological recovery

Questionnaire Item	Disability			Time Point			Interaction
	Permanent	Temporary	F	1	2	F	F
According to you how much will you recover after treatment? (very less = 0, very much = 5)	3.68	4.43	8.29[b]	3.88	4.63	10.89[b]	0.00
How is it true that something which has to happen will happen (very less = 0, very much = 5)	1.46	1.70	2.41	1.76	1.39	3.42	1.71
What are your plans after recovery from accident? (rater's judgement on 5-point scale)	2.20	2.69	3.83	2.28	2.71	6.41[a]	4.67[a]
How much do you believe in making efforts for complete recovery? (very less = 0, very much = 5)	4.78	4.60	0.89	4.53	4.85	3.59	0.02
Positive attitude	3.43	3.70	0.72	3.46	3.07	1.910	0.37
Overall psychological recovery	3.11	3.42	2.69	3.18	3.48	3.87[a]	1.21

Note: Degrees of freedom for these *F* ratios were 1 and 38.
  [a]$p < 0.05$; [b]$p < 0.01$.

implies that as time passed, the patients tended to recover psychologically from the crisis.

To examine how consistent these various indices of psychological recovery were, Cronbach's alpha (α) was computed. It was 0.58 when all 5 items were taken. However, the alpha value was markedly higher ($\alpha = 0.79$) when the perceived control measure was dropped. It was further observed that though all the indices had positive correlation with the overall recovery score, the correlation with 'control measure' was very low. It can thus be concluded that perceived controllability is not a good index of psychological recovery. This measure was, therefore, deleted from the composite score of recovery.

The correlations of causal attributions with psychological recovery were computed.

Table 4.4:

Correlations between causal attributions and psychological recovery

Causal Attribution	Temporarily Disabled		Permanently Disabled		Total Sample[a]
	Time 1	Time 2	Time 1	Time 2	
Karma	0.11	0.39[b]	0.43[b]	0.29[b]	0.37[b]
Own carelessness	0.08	0.30[b]	0.33[b]	0.01	0.18
Others' carelessness	0.08	0.11	0.16	0.25	0.05
Situation	0.16	−0.06	0.16	−0.14	0.02
Chance	−0.28	−0.05	0.09	−0.18	0.01
God's will	−0.08	−0.05	0.48[b]	0.29[b]	0.24

[a]Data across two time points were merged.
[b]$p < 0.10$.

Table 4.4 presents these correlations for the two groups. Correlations in Table 4.4 reveal that for the temporarily disabled patients at Time 1 the chance factor had significant negative correlation with recovery, that is, the more they attributed the accident to chance factor the less their recovery was. At Time 2, the recovery positively correlated with attribution to Karma and own carelessness. Permanently disabled patients showed a significantly high relation between recovery and attribution to Karma and God's will at both time points. Also at Time 1, attribution to own carelessness correlated with psychological recovery. The rest of the attributional categories did not relate to recovery. In general, merging data across two time points, only attribution to Karma was found correlated (positively) with psychological recovery.

The recovery index was also correlated with the doctor's assessment of the patients.

Table 4.5 reveals that, in general, when data of all the patients were taken after merging predominantly made to God's wish and chance factor. In many other studies conducted on samples from the Indian population, the poor (Sinha et al., 1980), the disadvantaged (Misra and Misra, 1986) and the depressed (Jain, 1987) very frequently made attributions to these factors for their lot. Hindus seem to be more inclined to attribute undesirable outcomes to external and uncontrollable factors. Findings on different religious groups are at variance. For example, Meyerowitz's (1980) strongly Catholic working class sample frequently attributed cancer to God's will, whereas Taylor et al.'s (1984) predominantly Jewish and upper middle class sample rarely did. The general point is that

Table 4.5:

Correlation between doctor's assessment and psychological recovery

Doctor's Assessment	Temporarily Injured		Permanently Injured		Total Sample
	Time 1	Time 2	Time 1	Time 2	
Severity of injury	−0.33[a]	0.15	0.19	0.21	0.22
No. of complaints	0.06	−0.14	−0.22	−0.05	−0.40[a]
Cooperation in treatment	−0.10	−0.00	0.08	−0.12	−0.01
Depressive symptoms	−0.08	−0.36[a]	−0.42[a]	−0.53[a]	−0.58[a]
Willingness to recovery	0.02	−0.15	0.08	−0.26	−0.05

[a] $p < 0.10$.

cultural and social factors render certain kinds of causal explanations more likely.

Another finding which deserves mention is the positive correlation between attribution to Karma and psychological recovery. Though attribution to this factor was not very high, this belief played a positive role in coping with the crisis. Belief in the principle of Karma is all pervasive among Hindus. For them this principle provides ready explanation for most of the happenings in life and is frequently invoked by the social support group. The attribution to Karma also reinforces one's faith in a just world. Bulman and Wortman (1977) in their study of patients with spinal cord injuries, found that those who were able to maintain their view of a just world despite their victimization, reported themselves to be happier than the other victims. In fact, the significant correlation between self-blame (own carelessness) and recovery is also consistent with faith in the just world and the theory of Karma.

It is interesting to note that in response to an open-ended question, patients with permanent disability made higher attribution to external factors than those who had temporary disability. For internal attribution, the case was just the reverse. From the controllability point of view, this implies that personal control is generally preferred when the outcome is temporary and modifiable, but not when the individual is confronted with a permanent, unmodifiable outcome. This finding supports the hypothesis of Bulman and Wortman (1977). Overall, the findings related to perceived control are equivocal. Contrary to the expectations, none of the three items of direct measure of controllability correlated with recovery. However, attribution to Karma implying perceived uncontrollability, and to own carelessness, indicative of perceived controllability, were associated with psychological recovery. Again, when asked about the factors contributing to recovery, almost 50% referred to God's will (uncontrollable). One possibility is that these contradictions in the findings reveal contradictions in the thinking of the accident victims, who were caught in the dilemma to have personal control or to forgo it. The findings ought to be seen in the light of harsh realities in which the patients were trapped. In the government hospital and other nursing homes, the facilities for treatment were very inadequate. Most of the victims were not economically well off to bear the burden of expensive treatment. They had little options to choosing doctors or the place of treatment. In this backdrop, the dilemma for the patients seems to be genuine.

However, the patients did not show the symptoms of learned helplessness. The findings showed that many temporarily disabled patients referred willpower as a contributing factor to recovery and were interested to inquire about the nature of treatment and duration of recovery. The permanently disabled victims were more interested in searching a meaning in their plight (attribution to Karma) and in asking the doctor about the duration and degree of recovery. These may be attempts at having interpretive and predictive secondary control (Rothbaum et al., 1982).

The other possibility is that the victims lacked concern to control the outcome and accept it as it comes. This could be symptomatic of the detachment which is highly valued and frequently preached in India. In an exploratory study, Pande and Naidu (1986) noted that people high on effort orientation and low on outcome orientation (a manifestation of detachment) showed less strain in a crisis situation. Detached people do make efforts to recover, but do not show concern to have control over the outcome. The therapeutic value of detachment, however, is yet to be fully comprehended.

In conclusion, it can be stated that the present study has successfully identified some of the possible correlates of psychological recovery. In reality there could be a vast variety of potential predictors in different crisis situations. What has fascinated the authors is the complexity and immense research possibilities in this emerging area. The findings have yielded many alternate hypotheses which could be explored in future research.

5

Health Beliefs and Psychological Adjustment to a Chronic Illness*

Putting up with a long-term disease not only involves physical discomfort but also creates many psychological problems for the patients. How people psychologically adjust to a chronic illness has been of interest in many recent studies (Burish and Bradley, 1983; Felton and Revenson, 1984; Reid, 1984; Taylor et al., 1984). The findings suggest that causal beliefs of the patients play an important role in coping and adjusting to a large variety of illnesses. Beliefs about what caused the disease help patients in deciding whether they should seek control or relinquish control to their health-care providers. Nicassio et al. (1985), for example, found in the case of arthritis patients that those who believed in personal control over the illness were less depressed and anxious, and exhibited less impairment in daily living.

The present study extends this line of investigation in two directions in the Indian cultural setting. First, along with causal, recovery beliefs were also examined. Recovery beliefs are the beliefs about the factors which

* Reprinted with permission from Dalal, A.K. and Singh, A.K. (1992). Role of causal and recovery beliefs in psychological adjustment to a chronic disease. *Psychology and Health: An International Journal, 6*, 193–203.

Dr Atul Kumar Singh is Reader in Psychology, Allahabad Degree College, University of Allahabad, Allahabad. This text has been edited for typographical errors, stylistic consistency, and sequential organization in order to make it suitable for inclusion in this book.

would contribute to physical recovery from the disease. Brickman et al. (1982) postulated that people do make a distinction between attribution of responsibility for the problem and responsibility for its solution. For example, one may consider oneself responsible for an illness but may consider doctor as responsible for recovery (or non-recovery) from the illness. Though the role of recovery beliefs had not been directly investigated in the earlier work, Affleck et al. (1987) found that negative mood was associated with the belief that health-care providers have greater control over the patient's daily symptoms. Since hospitalized patients are primarily concerned with the physical recovery, in the present study we hypothesized that their recovery beliefs would be more closely associated with perceived control and adaptational outcomes, than the causal beliefs. Secondly, we categorized causal and recovery factors as internal, external and cosmic in this study. In earlier investigations, cosmic factors (e.g. God, fate, Karma) had either not been considered, or were not treated as a separate category. In the Indian cultural setting, cosmic beliefs are presumed to be important determinants of all happenings in life, including sickness and suffering. The present study explored the role of cosmic beliefs in the psychological adjustment to a chronic disease.

A number of studies suggest that people do search for the causes of negative and unexpected outcomes (Weiner, 1985; Wong and Weiner, 1981). In a study by Greenberg et al. (1984), diabetic patients rated the causes of the illness as one of the most critical pieces of information from their physician at the time of diagnosis. Most of the patients reported perceived causes of their illness when questioned at any time point following their diagnosis. However, the frequency of the causes reported varied with the nature and severity of the disease. For example, lung cancer patients less frequently reported the causes of their illness than myocardial infarction patients (Mumma and McCorkle, 1982). Bulman and Wortman (1977) found that, in general, those paraplegic patients who had causal explanations for their accidents were better adjusted than those who had none. Patients gave varied causal explanations but the causal categories most frequently considered in those studies were others, self, situation and chance.

The question as to which of these causal beliefs would influence psychological adjustment has been investigated in many western studies. Abramson et al. (1978) and Miller and Norman (1979) postulated that helplessness would occur when people perceive the undesirable event as uncontrollable and attribute it to stable-internal causes (e.g. weak constitution). In a study of breast cancer patients, Taylor et al. (1984) found that blaming one-self (e.g. own-carelessness) was positively associated with superior coping. Self-blame implies taking personal responsibility for the illness, and could be indicative of regaining some sense of personal control. Consistent with this reasoning, attribution of blame to another person was associated with poor adjustment (Taylor et al., 1984). With arthritis patients, Affleck et al. (1987) found that perceiving greater personal control over one's medical care and treatment was associated with positive mood and psychosocial adjustment. There are, however, studies which did not find a positive relationship between dispositional self-blame and adjustment (Janoff-Bulman and Lang-Gunn, 1986; Major et al., 1985).

These health beliefs prevalent in the west have their basis in modern scientific medicine, where professional clinicians are the major source of explanations meaningful to the patients and their families. Whereas western explanatory models focus on curing the disease, most of the health beliefs in eastern cultures are concerned with healing, that is, attending to psychosocial needs of the patients (Carstairs and Kapur, 1976; Kleinman et al., 1978). The indigenous healing practices of the east emphasize supernatural causality, including punishment from sorcery, spirit or God (Joshi, 1988; Weiss et al., 1986). Folk religions in traditional societies of Asia structure beliefs about illness, choice of treatment alternatives and expectations from health practitioners. God's will (or deity) is presumed to play an important role in the recovery process. Many temples and shrines acquire great reputations for healing. In Buddha and Hindu traditions, another cosmic belief, the belief in Karma is widely accepted as a causal explanation for all major happenings in life. This concept implies that good and bad deeds accumulate over all previous lives and if people are suffering, they must have done bad deeds in this or in previous births (Gokhale, 1961; Paranjpe, 1984). Thus, when misfortune occurs, people attribute it to their own Karma, viewing themselves as causal agents in the metaphysical sense, as opposed to attribution to God's will and fate which impute no causal responsibility to the victim. In Ayurveda (the traditional Indian system of medicine) cosmic beliefs are interwoven in the scientific content. 'The *Carak Samhita* (one of the main texts for Ayurveda) ... talks of diseases resulting from the action of previous lives and the futility of curative efforts till the effects of individual Karma have been exhausted after taking their own pre-determined course' (Kakar, 1982, p. 225). Though Kakar argued that these cosmic principles are superimposed, they do constitute an Indian world-view of the causes of illness.

Dalal and Pande (1988) studied the role of causal beliefs in the psychological recovery of hospitalized accident victims with tempo-rary and permanent disability. Patients were interviewed one week and three weeks after the accident. It was found that attribution to Karma and one's own carelessness significantly correlated with psychological recovery of permanently disabled individuals on both the time points, whereas only on the second time point in the case of the temporarily disabled. God's will correlated with the psychological recovery only in the case of permanently disabled patients. Other attributional categories did not correlate with psychological recovery. It was suggested that when the outcome is not modifiable, belief in Karma and God's will moder-ate the feeling of bitterness and restores one's faith in the just world. Curiously, attribution to one's own carelessness (which implies personal control) also augmented the recovery process. The present study tested the veracity of these findings in the case of a chronic disease, where the outcome is modifiable.

Control related beliefs were also studied, in which a distinction was made between control over self and control over situation, as suggested by Rothbaum et al. (1982). According to Rothbaum et al., people often attempt to gain control by shaping existing physical, social and behavioural realities (termed as primary control). But on many occa-sions people resort to secondary control by leaving the existing unde-sirable realities unchanged by exerting control over their psychological consequences. This was termed as control over self by Rothbaum et al. Thus, whereas Rotter's theory of locus of control (Rotter, 1966) refers to general expectancies about life outcomes, Rothbaum et al. empha-size whether control efforts are directed to change self or to change the situation. It is still open to investigation as to how such control related beliefs are associated with psychological adjustment. Reid (1984) sug-gested that while facing serious chronic illnesses, patients try to balance their need to maintain a sense of mastery over their lives with their need to surrender the treatment of their disease to their health-care providers.

The present study was conducted on tuberculosis patients. Tubercu-losis is one of the least studied chronic diseases in terms of psychological adjustment, though it is one of the most frequently reported diseases in India. Statistics reveal that around 2% of the Indian population (about 15 million people) suffers from this disease at some stage in their life (Gill, 1977). According to the national survey (Health Information India, 1988), the mortality rate among hospitalized patients was 1.03% in 1987. There are no data as to how many patients die outside government hospitals. As a contagious, chronic disease tuberculosis creates several adjustment problems for patients. It is thus important to examine how far the existing knowledge about the factors contributing to psychological adjustment is generalizable to tuberculosis patients.

Method

Sample

Seventy Hindu male patients, hospitalized with a diagnosis of chest tuberculosis participated in the study. These patients were receiving treatment at two government hospitals affiliated with the Department of Chest Diseases and Tuberculosis of the M.L.N. Medical College, Allahabad. The sample constituted roughly 10% of the total in-patients, randomly selected from the hospital records. Of these patients, 38, 20 and 12 were from a rural, urban and semi-urban background, respectively, as noted from the records. The semi-urban individuals were those who had their house and family in the village but were working in a city. These patients were predominantly from lower castes and belonged to lower and lower-middle socio-economic strata, engaged in jobs such as office attendant, labour, agriculture, primary school teacher and small trader. As far as their education was concerned, 36 patients were illiterate, 12 were semi-literate (less than five years of formal education) and 22 were literate. The age of these patients varied from 16 to 70 years, with a mean age about 36 years. The average duration of their disease was about three years; it was less than one year for 32 patients, whereas for remaining 38 patients the duration of disease varied from 1 to 12 years. The mean severity ratings (on a 5-point scale) of the disease as reported by the patients and the doctors were 3.60 and 3.47, respectively, implying that the condition of the patients was perceived as moderately severe.

Questionnaire

A questionnaire in Hindi contained items from three domains: (a) information about the history of illness and treatment, (b) measures of causal and recovery beliefs, and (c) measures of perceived control and psychological adjustment. The first few items were related to the disease itself: history and nature of the disease, frequency of complaints, remedial steps taken and progress of the treatment.

The next set of questions was about causal attributions. The first item was an open-ended question asking patients to mention factors that they thought were responsible for their disease. The patients were then asked to rate six different causes to indicate the extent to which these were responsible for the illness. These causes were rated on a 5-point scale, having anchor points as 'least responsible' (1) and 'most responsible' (5). The other two items measured control over mind and disease, which refer to control over self and situation, respectively, according to Rothbaum et al.'s (1982) categorization. These items were: 'How much control do you have over your mind? and 'To what extent it would have been possible for you to avert this disease?' (English translation). These items were rated on a 5-point scale, on which one implied 'very little' and five implied 'very much.' Questions next in order were about the factors which might contribute to the recovery from the illness. Eight factors were rated by the patients for their possible contribution to their recovery, along a 5-point scale with end-anchors as 'very high contribution' (5) and 'very low contribution' (1).

The last set of questions was related to the psychological adjustment. Based on the review of various indices of good adjustment by Silver and Wortman (1980), three indices taken in this study were feeling of distress, hope and perceived severity of the illness. These were single-item measures on a 5-point scale and the overall good adjustment implied low distress, high hope of recovery and low rating of severity.

Procedure

The patients were contacted individually during their hospitalization. They were told about the purpose of the study and were assured that their answers would in no way influence their treatment in the hospital.

The patients were asked questions in a pre-assigned order, in a face-to-face interview. The responses were recorded verbatim. As a large number of patients were illiterate, care was taken to make them understand the rating scales. The interview took about 30 to 40 minutes per patient.

Finally, the doctors attending the patients were contacted and were asked to rate the severity of the illness of the patient on a 5-point scale, and also to assess expected recovery period.

Results

Causal Beliefs about the Disease

When asked to state the possible causes of their disease, 56 patients (80%) mentioned causes, though very few of them stated more than one cause. Content analysis of these causal descriptions revealed that own carelessness was mentioned by 16% of the patients. Other frequently reported causes were inadequate diet (11%), strenuous work routine (9%), unhygienic practices (7%), addiction (6%) and poverty (6%). The remaining causes were very specific and could not be categorized. Some such causes were loss of blood, punishment from the family deity, free-mixing with untouchables (lower caste) and getting injuries in an accident.

The patients also rated six given causes for the extent of responsibility for their disease. A one-way repeated measure analysis of variance across six causal factors was found significant ($F(5, 345) = 4.78$, $p < 0.01$). The mean ratings on six causal factors (fate; own carelessness; other's carelessness; family conditions; God's will; Karma) were 2.61; 2.69; 1.30; 2.31; 3.60 and 2.87, respectively. Mean comparisons using the Neuman–Keuls method (Winer, 1971) further showed that patients attributed maximum responsibility to God's will for their disease. Next in order were attributions to Karma, own-carelessness and fate, which did not differ significantly among themselves. Other's carelessness was regarded least responsible for their disease.

While comparing responses to open-ended items and rating-type items, discrepancies were found. Whereas cosmic factors were not frequently mentioned in response to an open-ended item, their mean ratings on a 5-point scale were high. To check whether or not the patients understood the attribution measure correctly, attribution to own-carelessness was correlated with the measure of self-blame, also included in the questionnaire. The correlation was found to be very high ($r = 0.63$, df = 68, $p < 0.01$), which indicates the validity of the attribution measure, particularly on the own-carelessness factor. In a post-hoc inquiry, many patients stated that they did not mention cosmic factors in the first instance, as they thought such causes to be too obvious to the researcher to inquire about. Some patients were hesitant to mention cosmic factors to an urban, educated researcher, particularly in the hospital setting.

To compare causal attributions for the disease across the three educational groups, we computed a one-way analysis of variance on rating scores. For none of the six causal factors was the F ratio significant, suggesting that education did not affect causal beliefs in this case.

Recovery Beliefs

Mean ratings on the eight recovery factors (self; God; family: doctor; fate; worship; money; Karma) were 2.59; 4.07; 2.43; 4.59; 3.29; 2.59; 3.21; 2.49, respectively. One-way repeated measure ANOVA was found significant ($F(7, 483) = 5.73$; $p < 0.01$). Mean comparisons further revealed that doctor and then God were regarded as the most important factors for recovery. Self, family, worship and Karma were considered as less important. Correlational analysis showed that only God, as a contributing factor, was associated with the severity judgment of the doctor ($r = 0.27$, df = 68, $p < 0.05$), that is, when the disease was more severe, God was believed as contributing more to the recovery.

To examine the effect of duration of illness on causal and recovery beliefs, patients were divided in two groups: those who had been ill for less than one year ($n = 32$) and those who had been ill for more than one year ($n = 38$). Differences were observed only in attributing the disease to other's carelessness ($F(1, 68) = 10.27$, $p < 0.01$). In this, patients who had been ill for less than one year, attributed the disease more to others ($M = 1.60$) than those who had been ill for more than one year ($M = 1.05$). Among the recovery beliefs, fate was less frequently considered to contribute by patients who had been ill for less than one year ($M = 2.91$) as compared with those who had been ill for more than one year ($F(1, 68) = 8.47$, $p < 0.01$). For other causal and recovery beliefs duration of illness was not an important factor.

Beliefs and Psychological Adjustment

The overall psychological adjustment score was obtained combining the scores along three indices, namely perceived severity, hope and distress. The Cronbach α for the combined score was 0.67. Since this value is just moderately high, analysis was done by taking these three indices separately, as well as taking a combined score. Table 5.1 shows the correlation of causal and recovery beliefs with perceived control and psychological adjustment.

Table 5.1:
Correlations of perceived control and psychological adjustment with causal and recovery beliefs

	Perceived Control		Psychological Adjustment			
	Mind	*Disease*	*Perceived Severity*	*Hope*	*Distress*	*Overall*
Causal beliefs						
Fate	−0.09	−0.29**	−0.10	−0.20	−0.13	−0.17
Own carelessness	0.10	0.54**	0.19	0.07	0.23	0.22
Others' carelessness	0.05	0.15	−0.25*	−0.13	−0.20	−0.26*
Family conditions	−0.01	0.03	−0.21	−0.16	−0.19	−0.24*
God's will	−0.18	−0.21	−0.11	−0.10	−0.16	−0.16
Karma	−0.23	−0.21	0.01	−0.23	−0.11	−0.12
Recovery beliefs						
Self	−0.21	0.40**	0.07	0.13	0.03	0.09
God	−0.43**	−0.13	−0.26*	−0.03	−0.33*	−0.29*
Family	−0.02	0.20	−0.01	0.15	−0.06	0.01
Doctors	0.13	0.12	−0.19	0.06	−0.003	−0.07
Fate	−0.19	0.07	−0.22	−0.19	−0.25*	−0.28*
Worship	−0.35**	0.06	−0.02	−0.08	−0.21	−0.14
Money	−0.02	0.12	−0.06	−0.003	−0.06	−0.06
Karma	−0.38**	−0.04	−0.002	−0.06	−0.16	−0.09
Doctor's report						
Severity of the disease	−0.04	−0.15	−0.46**	−0.14	−0.33*	−0.42**
Expected recovery	−0.07	0.10	0.20	0.17	0.14	0.22

Note: For the measures of psychological adjustment, high scores imply less perceived severity, high hope and less distress.
*$p < 0.05$, **$p < 0.01$.

Table 5.1 shows that none of the causal categories correlated with perceived control over mind, whereas only attribution to fate and own-carelessness correlated with perceived control over the disease. These correlations indicate that when the disease was attributed less to fate and more to one's own-carelessness, the perceived control over the disease was higher. Recovery beliefs appeared to be more closely associated with perceived control over mind than the causal beliefs. When the recovery was considered as contingent on God, worship and Karma, then less control over mind was perceived. The recovery belief in self had a positive correlation with perceived control over the disease.

As far as the overall psychological adjustment is concerned, causal attribution to external factors (other's carelessness and family conditions) negatively correlated with adjustment. In particular, attribution to other's carelessness correlated negatively with perceived severity. Again, when the cosmic factors (God and fate) were perceived as responsible for the recovery, psychological adjustment was poor. Specifically, the recovery factor God, correlated negatively with perceived severity and distress, whereas recovery factor fate correlated only with distress. No other causal and recovery factors were significantly associated with the psychological adjustment.

As regards control related beliefs, overall psychological adjustment had a significant association with perceived control over the disease ($r(68) = 0.24$, $p < 0.05$), but not with perceived control over mind. This suggests that when patients perceived more control over their disease, their psychological adjustment was better. Taken separately, indices of psychological recovery did not correlate with perceived control.

The doctor's report of the severity of the disease did not correlate with perceived control but was negatively correlated with overall psychological adjustment, particularly with perceived severity. The doctor's assessment of expected recovery correlated with the severity judgement ($r(68) = -0.41$, $p < 0.01$) but not with the patient's ratings of control and adjustment.

Discussion

The mean ratings of beliefs about causal and recovery factors revealed that patients attributed the causes of tuberculosis to God's will and Karma, whereas recovery was attributed to the doctor and God. In earlier work,

Dalal and Pande (1988) also found that the accident victims attributed their misfortune more to God's wishes than to any other factor. Attributing disease to God's will and Karma makes sense in a culture where religion pervades all life domains. Whenever people are in crisis, even the care-givers (e.g. family members) refer to these beliefs to explain the suffering, and subsequently, any recovery is attributed to God. Studies in other cultural settings have found supportive, as well as, non-supportive data on this causal category. For example, Meyerowitz's (1980) catholic working class sample frequently attributed cancer to God's will, whereas Taylor et al.'s (1984) predominantly Jewish upper-middle class sample rarely did. A cultural difference hypothesis may thus be proposed in causal beliefs about undesirable happenings.

In many traditional Asian countries such as China and India, beliefs in the contribution of cosmic factors to recovery are shared by folk practitioners and patients. Thus, for many chronic problems, patients reported greater improvement after consulting folk practitioners than modern physicians (Kakar, 1982; Kleinman and Sung, 1979). In India, for example, the Ayurvedic theory of epidemics affirms that many epidemics are inflicted by deities angered by the improper behaviour of local leaders (Weiss et al., 1986). In their study of an Indian village, Carstairs and Kapur (1976) noted that the traditional healers work on the principle that all problems of the patients are the results of misdeeds of the previous lives, committed by the suffering persons or their close kins. Many patients in the present study admitted in an informal chat that they did approach traditional healers (like Ojha, Holyman, Tantric, Pir), besides consulting a medical doctor. There was a general reluctance to admit this fact in a formal interview since such practices were thought to be incongruous with western style hospital setting.

It may be pointed out that in the present study Karma was considered as an important causal, but not a recovery factor by the patients. Such beliefs are consistent with the principle of Karma. This principle is supposed to explain what has already happened or is happening, but not what is going to happen (Gokhale, 1961). According to this principle, future events are supposed to be contingent upon several factors, including the individual's own efforts, besides Karma. The patients believed 'doctors' to be one of such important factors. It is quite likely that the hospital setting in which the patients were interviewed strengthened this belief. As noted by Krantz (1980) and Kornfeld (1972), hospitalization in itself constitutes a stressful event for most people, and many hospital procedures, viewed as routine by the staff, are anxiety provoking experiences for most patients. Thus, in a hospital setting, doctors are likely to be viewed by patients as the most powerful people, on whom they are totally dependent for recovery from the disease.

Interestingly, God's will and Karma as causal factors did not correlate with psychological adjustment. It appears that though such cosmic beliefs about the chronic illness are more frequently expressed in a particular cultural context, they do not necessarily (or directly) relate to the psychological adjustment. This finding is consistent with the one obtained in an earlier study (Dalal and Pande, 1988) on temporarily disabled patients. Thus, when the outcome is modifiable, as in the case of tuberculosis also, attributions to cosmic factors have little relevance, as far as psychological adjustment is concerned.

In general, it was found that the belief in external causal factors (other's carelessness and family conditions) were associated with low adjustment. Blaming other people and family conditions for the disease has implication in terms of the social support which a person needs in crisis. Such social support can protect the person against the stresses emanating from the illness, both physical and psychological, and creates a positive emotional state (Cobb, 1976). The findings of the present study do not support the inference of Taylor et al. (1984), in a study of breast cancer patients, that self-blame (own-carelessness) was positively associated with superior coping. However, this inconsistency in the finding could be of little consequence as the correlation value just missed the level of significance.

The recovery beliefs of a cosmic nature (God and fate) were associated with poor adjustment. This finding was somewhat unexpected, as religious people are generally thought to show better adjustment in a crisis situation. People experiencing tragic outcomes are frequently told by a support group to have greater faith in God (Dalal, 1988). In fact, the correlational nature of the data renders the task of interpreting the present finding a difficult one. A tentative explanation could be that those who believed that their recovery depended on cosmic factors saw little meaning in the hospital regimen and found the hospital environment as anxiety provoking. This explanation is consistent with Kleinman et al.'s (1978) observation that folk practitioners are more effective as far as healing is concerned. Again as stated by Bulman and Wortman (1977), chronic disease victims often experience a gradual process of breakdown, unlike accident victims who are normal one moment and injured the next. Fighting against a disease for a long period without success might induce a feeling of helplessness and a cynical view that the hospitalization and treatment is not going to work. However, before any attempt is made to fit the present finding in any theoretical framework, more empirical support is needed. In sum, though the hypothesis that recovery beliefs are more closely associated with psychological adjustment was not supported in a hospital setting, it did justify the distinction between causal and recovery beliefs as maintained in this study.

It was found that perceived control over the disease, but not over the mind, correlated with psychological adjustment. This finding is consistent with those obtained in studies of other chronic illness such as arthritis (Affleck et al., 1987) and coronary heart disease (Bar-On, 1984). The findings support the hypothesis that recovery beliefs have a closer relationship with perceived control than the causal beliefs. In fact, only one causal factor (i.e. own carelessness) had a significant and positive relation with perceived control over the disease. In the case of beliefs about the recovery factors, cosmic factors (God, worship and Karma) were linked with low perceived control over mind, whereas external factors (family and money) were associated with low perceived control over the situation. In a number of earlier studies (e.g. Bulman and Wortman, 1977), self-blame was found to be associated with a high sense of control over one's surroundings. A causal path may be hypothesized in which cosmic recovery beliefs lead to a low sense of personal control which in turn results in poor psychological adjustment. Future work should focus on testing this causal model in other cultural settings.

6

Beliefs about the World and Recovery from Myocardial Infarction*

How do people react to a major life crisis, such as myocardial infarction (MI), a technical term for heart attack, depends largely on the theories and beliefs they have about the world and about their disease. These beliefs, which are part of the broader socio-religious belief system that is prevalent in their culture, provide an understanding of the cause of the illness and of the factors that are likely to contribute to recovery. Wortman (1983) posited that patients' beliefs about the world play an important role in shaping their reactions to the sudden onset of a disease or disability, and influence the subsequent recovery process. On the basis of empirical work with hospital patients, Roberts et al. (1984) concluded that patients' beliefs about their health and treatment influence their behaviour much more than doctors or medical information do. Despite such convincing findings, there have been few attempts to examine the role of various beliefs in recovery.

One such belief, frequently reported in Western research, is the belief in a just world (Lerner, 1975). This belief has been found to influence people's reactions to a large variety of life events. The just world hypothesis refers to the belief that we live in a just world in which people get

* Agrawal, M. and Dalal, A.K. (1993). Beliefs about the world and recovery from myocardial infarction. *Journal of Social Psychology, 133*, 385–394.

Professor Manju Agrawal is Director, School of Social Science, Amity University, Lucknow. This text has been edited for typographical errors, stylistic consistency, and sequential organization in order to make it suitable for inclusion in this book.

what they deserve and deserve what they get (Lerner). According to this belief, if one performs good deeds, good outcomes will eventually follow. Such an assumption is essential if optimism and faith in good deeds are to be sustained. In their study of severe accident victims, Janoff-Bulman and Wortman (1977) found that those patients who were able to maintain their view of a just world despite the tragedy reported being happier than those patients who did not subscribe to such a belief. Janoff-Bulman and Wortman suggested that the belief in a just world and consequent self-blame made victims feel that the accident was avoidable and could be prevented in the future. However, this finding was not supported by other studies. Taylor et al. (1984) found no simple relationship between self-blame and adjustment among breast cancer patients. Instead, their findings revealed that self-blame was adaptive at some stages of recovery from the disease but not at others.

An Eastern counterpart of the just world belief is the doctrine of Karma, which extends the concept of justice to other worlds and other-births, implying a cumulative accounting of good and bad deeds in all previous lives. Accordingly, in this life one reaps what one has sown in one's previous lives (Radhakrishnan, 1926). The doctrine also proposes that every person is responsible for his or her own well-being and suffering. Blaming the self for suffering is integral to this principle, although this blame is in terms of causal responsibility, not moral responsibility (Gokhale, 1961; Paranjpe, 1984). The person absolves himself or herself from the guilt of having performed bad deeds because the doer of the deeds was a self of whom the person is not aware (Gokhale, 1961; Paranjpe, 1984). Karma, which is very widely accepted in India, not only restores one's faith in a just world but also provides a convincing explanation for a host of undesirable life events.

The influence of belief in Karma on the recovery of hospital patients in India has been examined in two studies. Dalal and Pande (1988) studied accident victims during their hospitalization and found that the attribution of an accident to Karma was positively correlated with the psychological of the patients, more so in the case of permanently disabled patients. In the second study (Dalal and Singh, 1992), belief in Karma was not significantly correlated with the psychological adjustment of hospitalized tuberculosis patients. One might conclude from these findings that belief in Karma will lead to different psychological outcomes, depending on the nature of the health impairment. In Western studies also, belief in life after death has been found to have a significant impact on adaptation to some life crises. Ulmer et al. (1989), for example, found that people who strongly believed in an afterlife recovered better, had a sense of well-being, and less actively avoided thinking about the death of their loved ones than those who did not strongly believe in an afterlife.

Belief in God, around which many other beliefs about the world are clustered, is frequently invoked in a crisis situation and differs significantly from the doctrine of Karma. In Karma, each individual is considered the causal agent for all pleasant and unpleasant happenings in his or her life. There are justified rewards and punishments for one's deeds in this life and in previous lives. In contrast, God is seen as an external agent who rewards and punishes, but not necessarily in accordance with what one deserves (Paranjpe, 1984). A person's bad deeds may be condoned by a benevolent God, who stands above the laws of the universe. Cross-cultural differences have been observed in the attribution of suffering to God. Whereas Meyerowitz's (1980) Catholic, working-class sample frequently attributed cancer to God's will, Taylor et al. (1984) predominantly Jewish, upper middle-class sample did so rarely. Hindu orthopedic patients (Dalal and Pande, 1988) considered God's wishes both as the cause of the accident and as a factor that was essential to recovery. However, the belief that God's wishes were a cause of the accident was significantly correlated with psychological recovery only when the disability was of a permanent nature. Despite the salience of belief in God in a crisis situation, researchers have not systematically examined the health-related consequences of such religious beliefs (Siegel, 1986).

In this study we compared the effect of different beliefs about the world on the recovery of MI patients. A distinction was made among world beliefs (cultural beliefs about the life and existence), causal beliefs (factors to which the patients attributed their sickness) and recovery beliefs (factors patients considered as the contributors to recovery). Although all beliefs are culturally rooted, world beliefs are relatively culture-specific and enduring, whereas causal and recovery beliefs are relatively situation specific.

Most studies have examined only causal attributions for health problems, (Weary et al., 1989) and have not distinguished among world, causal, and recovery beliefs. Brickman et al. (1982) argued that people do distinguish between attribution of responsibility for a problem and responsibility for its solution. For example, an MI patient may have a strong belief in God (world belief), may not hold God responsible for the infarction (causal belief), yet may think that his recovery depends on God's will (recovery belief).

We examined beliefs in a just world, God and Karma in the present research in the context of world, causal and recovery beliefs. Because considering the just world as causal and recovery beliefs did not seem reasonable, its corollary, self, was taken both as a causal and a recovery belief. Thus, we examined MT patients' world beliefs in a just world, Karma and God, and their causal and recovery beliefs one for self, Karma, and God. We expected that MI patients' beliefs in the three contexts (world, causal, and recovery) would differ and that, consequently, these beliefs would have a differential role in their recovery.

We measured both the physical and the psychological recovery of the MI patients. The attending doctors were asked to evaluate the physical recovery of the patients 4 to 5 days after they had been hospitalized for MI. We assessed the patients' psychological recovery by interviewing them at two time points, in the hospital setting, 4 to 5 days after the onset of the disease (Time 1), and in the home setting, about a month later (Time 2).

Method

Sample

The sample comprised 70 male, Hindu MI patients who were being treated at the Swaroop Rani Nehru Hospital in Allahabad. Their ages ranged from 35 to 65 years, with a mean of about 51 years, and they had an average income of 2,700 rupees (US$90) per month, which considered middle class. The subjects' average level of education was around high school. It was the first incidence of MI for all the patients, and all had stayed in the intensive coronary care unit for a minimum of 6 hours and a maximum of 4 days.

Interview Schedule

The interview, which was in Hindi, included items that pertained to belief in God, Karma, and a just world. Belief in God was measured by a single item, 'How much faith do you have in God?' Belief in Karma and a just world were measured by five items (alpha = 0.56) and four items (alpha = 0.63), respectively. Three of these items were derived from a measure of just world (Collins et al., 1973). The items were to be considered from the perspective of all previous births when belief in Karma was being measured and from the perspective of this birth only when belief in just world was being measured. For example, 'One reaps what one has sown in all previous births' was an item that measured belief in Karma, and 'One reaps what one has sown in this life' was the corresponding item that measured belief in a just world.

Causal attribution for MI to God, Karma and self were each measured by a single item. The patients' beliefs in the contribution of God, Karma, and self to their recovery were also measured by a single item each. All the items were measured on 5-point scales that ranged from *least* (1) to *utmost* (5) faith, causal responsibility or perceived contribution of God, Karma or just world/self.

The indices of psychological recovery were in terms of the patients' reports about the severity of the disease, expectation of recovery, perceived recovery and mood state. The indices were rated on 5-point scales, and the number of items ranged from three to six. Cronbach's alpha for these measures ranged from 0.67 to 0.81. The doctor's rating of the patients' physical recovery was in terms of each patient's progress (on a 5-point scale) since hospitalization. This assessment was made based on the clinical and biochemical data available to the doctor. Background information about the patients (e.g. age, education, income) was also noted.

Procedure

With the permission of the attending doctor, we interviewed the patients individually in the hospital on the 4th or 5th day after the onset of their disease. The patients initially responded to our queries about themselves and their disease. This helped us to establish a rapport. We then inquired about the patients' beliefs and psychological recovery. This interview took about 30 to 40 mm to complete. Sometimes we conducted an interview in two sessions if a patient reported exhaustion or unwillingness to continue. We also asked the attending doctor about the patient's physical recovery.

After a month, we again interviewed the patients, this time at their residence, about their recovery from MI.

Results

We computed the correlations of the demographic variables with the three categories of beliefs. Age, education, income and number of dependent children were correlated with the measures of beliefs. Only 3 out of a total of 36 correlations were significant; hence, it was deduced that these beliefs were quite pervasive, cutting across demographic boundaries. These results justified the non-partitioning of the MI patient sample along these demographic variables.

We computed the intercorrelations among the three categories of beliefs and found that world beliefs in God, Karma and a just world were significantly ($p < 0.01$) positively correlated with each other and with recovery beliefs for God, Karma and self (r ranged from 0.36 to 0.89). The recovery beliefs were also significantly correlated with each other (with the exception of recovery beliefs in God and self). These results suggested that the patients who had a strong world belief in God, Karma or just world also attributed a great part of their recovery to these agencies. In contrast, only a few causal beliefs were significantly intercorrelated. World beliefs in God and Karma were significantly correlated only with causal attribution to Karma ($r = 0.25$ and 0.34, respectively, $p < 0.01$), implying that the more strongly a person believes in God or Karma, the more he or she attributes to the power of Karma. Attributions to God and self were not correlated with any of the world beliefs and were negatively correlated with each other ($r = -0.39$, $p < 0.01$). Attribution to God was negatively correlated with recovery belief in Karma ($r = -0.40$, $p < 0.01$), whereas attribution to Karma was positively correlated with recovery belief in God ($r = 0.34$, $p < 0.01$).

The correlations of these three types of beliefs with various indices of the physical and psychological recovery of the MI patients are presented in Table 6.1. Because the patients' physical and psychological recovery depended on the severity of their MI, the doctors' ratings for the severity of MI were partialled out from the measures of recovery. Hence, the correlations in Table 6.1 are partial correlations. For two indices of recovery (perceived recovery and mood state) data were obtained at two time points. For the three other indices (perceived severity, expectation of recovery, and medical recovery), data were obtained only at the first time point. Because we measured these indices using multiple items,

Table 6.1:

Partial correlations of world, causal and recovery beliefs for physical and psychological recovery

Index of Recovery	Cronbach's Alpha	World Belief			Causal Belief			Recovery Belief		
		God	Karma	Just World	God	Karma	Self	God	Karma	Self
Time 1										
Medical recovery	–	-0.03	0.21	0.26*	-0.37**	-0.09	0.24*	0.31**	0.38**	0.15
Perceived severity	0.76	-0.13	0.22	-0.17	0.09	0.05	0.13	0.06	-0.14	0.14
Expectation of recovery	0.73	0.20	0.39**	0.48**	-0.22	0.09	0.16	0.29**	0.48**	0.41**
Perceived recovery	0.67	0.28*	0.34	0.37**	-0.23*	0.04	0.20	0.27*	0.49**	0.15
Positive mood	0.71	-0.3	-0.03	-0.2	-0.17	-0.01	0.03	-0.14	-0.15	0.01
Time 2										
Perceived recovery	0.81	-0.05	0.21	0.15	-0.37**	0.19	0.30**	0.29**	0.29**	0.24*
Positive mood	0.67	-0.18	0.13	0.11	-0.41**	0.07	0.32**	0.14	0.19	0.02

Note: We obtained partial correlations after partialling out the severity of the MI ratings from different indices of recovery. Except for physical recovery, which was based on the doctor's report, all data were obtained from the patients.

$^*p < 0.05$, $^{**}p < 0.01$.

we computed Cronbach's alpha for each index and found it to be reasonably high (see Table 6.1).

Table 6.1 indicates that the patients' physical recovery was significantly correlated with belief in a just world, and with recovery belief in God and Karma. The patients' physical recovery was negatively correlated with God and positively correlated with self, as causes of the illness, implying that those who attributed the cause to God did not recover as well as those who attributed the cause to self. The indices of psychological recovery, perceived severity and mood state were not correlated with any category of beliefs at Time 1. Expectation for recovery was associated with belief in Karma and a just world, as with all recovery beliefs, implying that the patients had a higher expectation for recovery when they had a strong belief in Karma and a just world and also considered each of (a) God, (b) Karma and (c) self as responsible for recovery.

Perceived recovery was significantly correlated with all three world beliefs at Time 1, but with none of them at Time 2; no index of recovery correlated with any of the world beliefs at Time 2. At both Time 1 and Time 2, perceived recovery was negatively correlated with the attribution of MI to God implying that the more the patients attributed cause to God, the weaker their perceived recovery. At Time 2, perceived recovery was positively correlated with self-blame (attribution to self). Again, perceived recovery was positively associated with the belief in the contribution of God and Karma at Time I and with all the three recovery beliefs, including self, at Time 2. Mood state was associated only with causal beliefs at Time 2, that is, positive mood state was associated with greater attribution to self and less attribution to God.

Discussion

Belief in God, Karma and a just world were pervasive among the Hindu patients in this study, cutting across the boundaries of age, socioeconomic status, family size and education. Although patients' degree of faith in God or Karma varied, the patients were rarely nonbelievers. This finding was not surprising because spirituality is emphasized from early childhood in the Indian culture (Carstairs, 1957).

The three world beliefs were significantly inter-correlated. In fact, as argued by many writers (e.g. Gokhale, 1961; Radhakrishnan, 1926), the belief in Karma subsumes beliefs in a just world and God and also extends the concepts of justice beyond this life, across all previous incarnations. In this scheme God is supposed to be imparting reward and punishment, according to some law. These beliefs about the world were closely associated with recovery beliefs but not with causal beliefs, suggesting that beliefs about the world predict the factors to which patients will attribute their recovery. In contrast, the causal beliefs had few significant correlations with world and recovery beliefs. By definition, causal beliefs are beliefs about the conditions that cause MI. Thus they are specific to a particular event and change as the appraisal of the event changes (Kelley, 1967). Beliefs about the world are part of an individual's general belief system and are relatively stable over time. The results of this study also justify the consideration of causal and recovery beliefs about MI as separate belief categories. Causal beliefs cannot be inferred on the basis of salient world and recovery beliefs. The distinction between causal and recovery beliefs has also been supported by a previous study (Dalal and Singh, 1992).

The patients' perception of the severity of their MI was independent of any of the beliefs we were studying. In previous Western research, a negative relationship was found between perceived severity and belief in a just world (Janoff-Bulman and Wortman, 1977). This relationship was not supported in the present study with Hindu patients. In a previous study (Dalal and Singh, 1992) on hospitalized tuberculosis patients, causal and recovery beliefs were not related to the perceived severity of the disease, and belief in Karma and a just world were associated with the expectation of recovery. Belief in Karma reaffirms one's faith in natural justice because Karma implies that positive deeds will lead to better outcomes. This contention is also consistent with belief in a just world.

The present study indicated that the three types of beliefs were related differently to recovery at Time 1 and Time 2. In general, world beliefs were positively associated with recovery from the disease at Time 1, and causal beliefs in God and self were significantly but negatively correlated with recovery at Time 2. Recovery beliefs were positively correlated with recovery at both Time 1 and Time 2.

The factor to which the patients attributed their disease was associated with their physical recovery. When the patients blamed God for their disease, they showed poor physical (doctor-assessed) and self-assessed recovery, and their mood was less positive. When the patients blamed themselves for the onset of MI, physical recovery was better, and there was a more positive perception of recovery and mood state at Time 2. As for the mechanism of causal attributions, the MI patients who blamed themselves for their disease may have developed a sense of control over the disease and its recurrence. The MI patients who attributed their illness to factors under their personal control have been found to initiate active efforts towards recovery from the disease and towards preventing recurrence of the disease, for example, by engaging in adaptive health behaviour (Bar-On, 1984). Efforts to enhance a sense of control in cardiac patients have been found in other studies to be beneficial (Cromwell et al., 1977). The Type A behaviour pattern, which is characterized by efforts to control stressful situations (Glass, 1976) but is considered a major risk factor for MI, has been associated with longer survival than has Type B behaviour (Ragland and Brand, 1988).

The more the MI patients recovered psychologically and physically, the more they credited God and Karma for their recovery. The patients attributed their recovery to self-effort only at Time 2. Because the initial period of MI is characterized by much anxiety and uncertainty, world beliefs and recovery beliefs in God and Karma may have given patients the inner strength to cope with the crisis, resulting in better physical and perceived recovery. Perhaps the patients needed time to regain a sense of personal control in order to initiate health-regulatory behaviour.

The present study has demonstrated that the patients' beliefs about their disease were closely linked with their recovery from MI. Although causal and recovery beliefs were measured by single items, many of the findings corroborated previous research with patients from the same cultural background (Dalal and Pande, 1988; Dalal and Singh, 1992). The results of this study suggest that the recovery of MI patients might be augmented by changing their beliefs about the world and about their illness.

7

Development of a Measure of Psychological Recovery

A major objective of the present study was to develop a verbal measure of psychological recovery of the patients who are hospitalized for a chronic problem. A scale measuring four different aspects of psychological recovery was prepared and validated on patients with myocardial infarction, cancer, abdominal surgery and orthopaedic problems. The demographic correlates of psychological recovery were also investigated.

Psychological recovery refers to patient's attitude towards his or her own disease or disability, which gets manifested in forms of restlessness, loss of appetite, sleeping disorder, stress and anxiety. These psychogenic symptoms aggravate the pain and discomfort due to the disease and retard recovery. The patients do not feel treated unless their psychological recovery keeps pace with physical recovery. Often psychological recovery is an important criterion for attending doctors and relatives to infer, whether or not, patient is responding to the medication. Doctors decide about the course of treatment not only on the basis of physical symptoms but also on the basis of reported discomfort and complaints of the patients. Frequently, a decision to discharge a patient is taken on the basis of patients' verbal report of feeling good and cured (Taylor, 2006).

Research in this area is accumulated on the basic assumption that the mind and the body are closely intertwined. A large number of physical diseases are caused by the chronic stresses. More importantly, body's healing mechanism works efficiently only when the patients can control their anxiety and have a positive orientation. Physical recovery is affected by the way patients mobilize their internal resources and preserve hope. Conversely, patient's psychological recovery is affected by their physical recovery. In this respect, the term psychological recovery is subsumed under the broader domain of mental health and psychological well-being.

A review of the available literature reveals that the term psychological recovery is used differently in different contexts. As a psychological response to physical health problems the terms that are often used interchangeably are sickness impact (Bergner et al., 1981), psychological adjustment (Taylor, 1984), successful coping (Silver and Wortman, 1980), acceptance (Kubler-Ross, 1969), common psychiatric symptoms (Langner, 1962) and general well-being (Smith and Ruiz, 2002). Consequently, there is a great deal of conceptual variations in the measures developed in this field. There are disagreements over the intent and conceptual interpretation of the scales (McDowell and Newell, 1987). The problem is exacerbated by the tendency of the authors of earlier scales not to provide operational definitions of 'what they were attempting to measure'. Most of the earlier scales were developed empirically, by selecting questions that distinguish between 'normal' and 'emotionally distressed' persons. This approach led to many interpretational problems. For example, widely used Langner's (1962) 22-item scale is said to be indicative of mental health, emotional adjustment, psychological disturbance, psychiatric or psychological symptoms and mental illness (Meile, 1972). Such disagreements render it difficult to empirically generalize the findings. Bergvik (2008) has referred various psychological factors that cause and constitute psychological recovery in case of heart diseases. Mital et al. (2004) considered return to work after a coronary heart problem as a strong indicator of psychological recovery.

Oftentimes, the term adjustment is used to denote patients' positive mental health and well-being in the face of a chronic health condition. The term 'adjustment' is also used to refer how well patients manage to live with the disease in different life domains. People vastly differ in how they cope and adjust to chronic health problems and their consequences. Stanton et al. (2001) posited that conceptualization of adjustment to a chronic disease include mastery of disease-related adaptive tasks, maintenance of daily activities, perceived quality of well-being, absence of psychological disorders and absence of negative mood state. These components of adjustment are, in fact, interrelated and at times difficult to be isolated.

Adjustment is rather an amorphous term, all-encompassing but without any clear directionality. Furthermore, adjustment connotes living with a disease, and does not give a clear sense of psychologically thriving in the disease condition, gaining a sense of mastery over one's affective and mental state. It is our contention that the term psychological recovery is more focused, positive and proactive. It rhymes with physical recovery and can be employed in the similar sense for evaluating affective, conative and action states, a kind of attitude which people have towards their health problem.

The term psychological recovery can be better understood in the light of its following attributes: One, psychological recovery is conceptualized as independent of the disease condition. A physical condition may stabilize or aggravate but psychological recovery may take its own course. People may be more composed and in control in deteriorating physical condition and can be more distressed even if there is physical improvement. Both are, indeed, equally important for better health status. Two, psychological recovery is not just overcoming the distress and uncertainty caused by the disease condition. A long-term disease results in many physical, social, relational and emotional disruptions in life and calls for major changes in everyday living. There is no way one can go back to the earlier mode of living and psychological recovery in this sense would imply regaining post-disease mode of psychological functioning. Three, psychological recovery is a dynamic process. Like in the case of physical recovery, psychological recovery also goes through many remissions and relapses. During the course of psychological recovery, the physical pain and suffering that one has undergone and lived with, can rarely be eradicated from one's psyche and its memory and apprehension keeps bothering the person. Fourth, psychological recovery does not follow any predictable path or stages. It is possible to develop a psychological measure of recovery but not much can be said about the course of psychological recovery, vis-à-vis physical recovery.

Some Forerunners of Psychological Recovery Measure

Some of the measures that were developed in the past are briefly presented here.

Millon Behavioral Health Inventory (MBHI) (Millon et al., 1979). It is a 150-item self-report questionnaire, organized into 20 subscales. These subscales are again arranged into four domains, which include (a) coping styles, (b) psychogenic attitudes, (c) psychosomatic complaints and (d) a prognostic index. The MBHI seeks to (a) describe the psychological styles of medical service recipients, (b) examine the impact of emotional and motivational needs and coping strategies on disease course and (c) suggest a comprehensive treatment plan to decrease the impact of deleterious psychological reactions.

Psychosocial Adjustment to Illness Scale (PAIS) (Derogatis, 1977; Derogatis and Lopez, 1983). The PAIS is a 46-item instrument designed to measure psychosocial adaptation to medical illnesses and chronic diseases. The scale can be administered both as a semi-structured psychiatric interview by a trained clinician and as a self-report measure (PAIS-SR). In addition to an overall adjustment score, seven subscales are provided. These include Health Care Orientation, Vocational Environment, Domestic Environment, Sexual Relationships, Extended Family Relationships, Social Environment and Psychological Distress (i.e. indicating reactions of anxiety, depression, guilt, and hostility, as well as levels of self-esteem and body image).

Acceptance of Disability (AD) Scale (Linkowski, 1971). The AD scale is a 50-item, six-point, summated rating scale developed to measure the degree of acceptance of disability as theorized by Dembo et al. (1956). Items are summed to yield a single score representing changes in one's value system following the onset of physical disability.

Sickness Impact Profile (SIP) (Bergner et al., 1976; Gilson et al., 1975). The SIP comprises 136 items that yield, in addition to scores on 12 subscales, a global scale score; three scales can be combined to create a physical dimension score. Weaknesses are suggested by scant concurrent validity data, lack of normative data across disabling conditions, and potential confounding effects of response bias influences.

Most of these measures are old and culture-specific. Furthermore, none of them are directly pertaining to the notion of psychological recovery and conceptualized herewith. Keeping this in view, a new measure of psychological recovery was prepared to be appropriate for Indian population.

Development of a Measure

In the present study, the term 'psychological recovery' is defined in rather a restricted sense of positive mental attitude, leading to successful coping. It is contended that a major chronic illness or accidental injury causes shock, confusion and disorientation for the victim, a feeling that the life is gone off balance. As the symptoms and subsequent problems become more pressing, people realize that their existing patterns of adjustment are inadequate. They experience a considerable degree of anxiety and stress. It takes them time to gradually return to a 'normal' level of functioning. Psychological recovery in this sense can be viewed as a process of returning to the state of mental functioning prior to the present crisis. Psychological recovery is thus viewed as an index of positive change in mental functioning over a period of time, in the same manner as physical recovery is a positive change in body conditions. As the body has its own built-in mechanism to repair and restore the body to the state prior to illness or injury, so is the mind's own mechanism to restore its prior mental state (Siegel, 1991).

What we still do not know is the nature of relationship between medical and psychological recovery, except that it is not an isomorphic one. For example, Stone et al. (1987) using daily diary method examined the relation between positive and negative mood states and antibody generation (carriers of immunity). They found that antibody level was higher on the days when respondents reported high positive mood state. These results were replicated in a subsequent study that monitored mood and antibody levels over a 12-week period (Stone et al., 1992). In a study of myocardial infarction patients, Agrawal and Dalal (1993) found a positive relationship between positive life orientation and adjustment to myocardial infarction. Fife (1994) concluded that what is more important is how patients construct the meaning of their illness and when they assign positive meanings, it has implications for their recovery from the illness.

The development of this measure of psychological recovery has relied on other existing measures. Bulman and Wortman (1977) used an open-ended measure of successful coping of the accident victims. Further reviewing the field, Silver and Wortman (1980) identified many characteristics indicative of successful coping and recovery. These include, keeping one's distress within manageable limits, maintaining a realistic appraisal of the situation, being able to function or carry out socially desired goals, maintaining a positive self-concept, and maintaining a positive outlook of the situation. A review of the more recent mental health, coping and strain measures suggest a wider net for measuring psychological recovery. The classical mental health measures (e.g. Caplan et al., 1986; Pande and Naidu, 1992) focused on physical and psychosomatic symptoms. The wide range of coping measures have covered specific aspects as hope, expectations, positive construction, appraisal of the illness condition, affective disorders, social interactional process, self-care, etc. These vast arrays of indices could be categorized into four domains: illness appraisal, psychosomatic symptoms, mood state and positive orientation. These four domains formed the basis for developing the psychological recovery measure in this study.

Various considerations prompted development of this new scale. First, no such measure existed in psychological literature that appraises recovery from patient's perspective. Patients' own report of their affective and cognitive state should be more reliable than the observational reports of attending doctors and relatives. The need for such a scale in the area of health research can hardly be overemphasized. Second, in all health problems it is desirable to monitor both the physical and psychological change processes. In research, only a mediated relationship is evidenced between psychological recovery and physical recovery. Such a measure is needed to establish the role of person and illness-related moderator variables. Third, such a measure should be of much help in studying self-healing process. Understanding the way a patient deals with the crisis, overcomes psychological traumas and mobilizes one's own internal resources over a period of time can give us an important understanding of how people recover from a crisis. Fourth, understanding the pace of psychological recovery of patients is necessary to make various treatment-related decisions. It is likely that a patient showing better psychological recovery would be more communicative and cooperative during hospitalization.

Method

Developing a Measure of Psychological Recovery

Psychological recovery scale went through various stages of development before its final version for data collection was prepared. At the initial stage, health professionals (doctors and nurses), clinical and academic psychologists and patients were asked open-ended questions about their own understanding of psychological recovery. Categories that repeatedly emerged in their responses were hope, perceived stress, positive mood state and self-care. In the second stage, items related to these categories were included in the initial measures of psychological recovery/adjustment in three studies, which are included in this book. Though these measures were forerunners of the present scale, they were found to be reliable measures of psychological recovery. The repeat administration of these measures evidenced that they were sensitive to record changes over a period of time.

To make the measure more exhaustive and psychometrically sound, the primary focus in the study was on preparing a full length measure and testing it out on a wide cross-section of patients. A comprehensive scale was prepared, which included items from the previous scales, as well as, from the responses obtained in an open-ended enquiry.

The scale had five sections. The first section was general enquiry about the demographic background of the patient and the history of the medical problem for which they were presently hospitalized. The next four sections were four subscales of the recovery measure, namely illness appraisal, psychosomatic symptoms, mood state and positive orientation.

The first subscale: illness appraisal had statements related to the patient's own evaluation of his or her illness and recovery, mostly in comparison to illness and recovery of other patients in similar conditions. The patients were asked 'to what extent the statements were true in their case (very less to very much)?' The second subscale: psychosomatic symptoms included those physical symptoms, which had psychological basis as well, like difficulty in breathing, insomnia and irritability. The patients rated the increased or decreased frequency of these symptoms after getting admitted to the hospital. The third subscale: mood state mapped their emotional state. It included those thoughts and anxieties, which they have while convalescing in the hospital. The feelings mentioned were like feeling of hopelessness, fear of doom and feeling hurt. The frequency of these feelings was rated in terms of never occurring to always occurring. The last subscale: positive orientation had items, which refer to positive construction of the illness, that is, whether or not patients find something positive in their experience of falling sick or getting injured. Such thoughts were rated in terms of agreement—from very much to very less. All the statements were rated on a 5-point scale.

There were a large number of items in the initial version of the scale. On the basis of pretesting, few items were eliminated. The criteria were: comprehensibility, frequency of actually occurring, relevance and repetition. In the administered version of the scale, there were 14 (8 positive, 6 negative), 8 (all negative), 26 (8 positive, 18 negative) and 8 (7 positive, 1 negative) items for the subscales of illness appraisal, psychosomatic symptoms, distress and positive orientation, respectively. The complete scale is given in Appendix A.

In addition, there was a two-item measure for the attending doctor to indicate overall recovery of the patients. Similarly, there was a six-item measure for the accompanying relative to indicate the overall recovery of the patient.

Sample

The psychological recovery scale was administered on 80 adult hospital patients. These patients were hospitalized either for abdominal surgery, myocardial infarction, cancer or orthopaedic injuries. There were an equal number of 20 patients in each category. The number of male and female patients was 54 and 26, respectively. In that, all heart patients were male as were all except one orthopaedic patient. Half of the cancer patients and one-third of the surgery patients were males. The age of these patients ranged from 20 to 65 years.

Most of these patients came from the rural area of Allahabad district, within a distance of 1 to 80 kilometres. The education of 75% of the patients was below high school, of which 24% had no formal education. Only four patients had education up to and above graduation. Most of the patients were in job (34%) or small business (20%), or were agriculturalists (26%). The income of 70% of the patients was below ₹2,000 per month. These patients were clearly from rural lower-middle class.

All these patients were getting treatment in the Swaroop Rani Hospital, a district government hospital located in Allahabad city. Most of these patients were in the hospital for about a week at the time of being first contacted. The duration of the sickness as reported by these patients was short (between 3 days and 4 weeks) for heart and orthopaedic problems and was longer in case of surgery and cancer (between 2 weeks and 3.5 years) patients. The facilities at this hospital were typical of a government free-service hospital and most patients found them far from satisfactory. Each patient was accompanied by at least one relative, mostly spouse, parents or grown-up children.

Data Collection

The patients were identified with the help of doctors on duty in the general wards of the Swaroop Rani Hospital where they were under treatment. Only those patients who were permitted by the attending doctors and relatives to talk were interviewed. Most of the patients were in the hospital for at least 4–5 days at the time of interviewing. Patients' prior consent was taken, and an appointment was fixed according to their convenience. The interviews were conducted by a research assistant who had a doctoral degree in psychology.

The psychological recovery scale was completed by the patients in a face-to-face interview situation. They were explained the five-point rating scale and it was ensured that they understood the instructions. The researcher read each item and the patients gave their response in terms of one of the five category points. All questions in the recovery scale were asked in a predetermined order. On an average, it took patients 25–30 minutes in completing the schedule. The scale was completed in one sitting; in few cases, it took two or three sittings when the patients were unwilling to continue for varied reasons.

The attending doctor and relative were also given a small questionnaire to complete about medical and overall recovery of the patients.

Seventeen of the 80 patients were re-interviewed after an interval of one week. These patients were randomly selected from those who were still in the hospital. This time they were given only psychological recovery scale.

Result

Item Analysis

Four criteria were considered for final selection of the items. These were standard deviation, item-total correlation, discrimination index and test–retest scores.

The pre-assigned criteria for a good item was high standard deviation (above 0.75), high item-total correlation (above 0.28), high t values indicating discrimination ($t > 2.88$) and high t value for test-retest mean scores ($t > 1.0$). These cut points were decided once the results were obtained. The items that conformed to at least three of the four criteria were retained.

Items in Appendix A that are marked with asterisk are those which are deleted from the final version. These are items 10 and 13 in the first, items 5 and 6 in the second, items 7 and 17 in third and item 7 in the fourth subscale, respectively.

Table 7.1 shows characteristics (mean, SD, α) of each subscale, as well as, of the overall psychological recovery scale. The Cronbach alphas (αs) for all, except third subscales ranged from 0.64 to 0.68, which are moderately high; the Cronbach alphas for both the third subscale and the overall scale were 0.90. It establishes that all subscales of psychological recovery are highly homogeneous.

The last two columns in Table 7.1 show the correlations of the subscales with doctor's and relative's assessment of the overall recovery of the patients. None of the subscales and overall scale had significant correlation with the doctor's ratings, implying that psychological recovery and doctor's assessment are independent and do not overlap. On the contrary, all subscales had significant positive correlations with the relative's assessment. It seems that relative's assessment was more on the lines of psychological assessment, whereas the doctor's assessment was more in terms of medical recovery. Again, correlation between

Table 7.1:

Mean, SD, Cronbach alphas (α) for all four subscales of psychological recovery and their correlations with doctor's and relative's ratings

| | No. of | | | | Correlations | |
Subscales	Items	Mean	SD	α	Doctor	Relative
Illness appraisal	12	3.29	0.46	0.66	0.12	0.42*
Psychosomatic symptom	6	2.27	0.58	0.64	0.01	0.37*
Mood state	24	3.47	0.69	0.90	0.06	0.57**
Positive orientation	7	3.89	0.59	0.68	0.04	0.30*
Overall	49	3.34	0.47	0.90	0.12	0.39*

Note: Mean values are on a 5-point scale.

*$p < 0.05$, **$p < 0.01$.

Table 7.2:
Intercorrelation among the subscales of psychological recovery (n = 80)

Subscales	1	2	3	4
1. Illness appraisal		0.41*	0.48*	0.35*
2. Psychosomatic symptoms			0.34*	0.15
3. Mood state				0.25
4. Positive orientation				
Overall	0.71*	0.52*	0.94*	0.47*

*$p < 0.01$.

doctor's assessment and relative's assessment was not statistically significant ($r = 0.21$, df = 78).

Table 7.2 shows the intercorrelations among the four subscales. Illness appraisal had significant correlations with all other subscales, whereas positive orientation did not correlate with the other two subscales. Psychosomatic symptoms and mood state significantly correlated with each other. All the subscales had significant correlations with the overall scale; mood state subscale having the highest whereas positive orientation the lowest one.

Shorter Versions of the Scale

Often there is a need to have a short version of the psychological recovery scale for quick appraisal. Looking at the psychometric properties of different subscales, it was found that mood state reaction subscale is best suited for this purpose. This subscale had very high ($r = 0.90$) correlation with the overall scale.

To have even a shorter version, the mood state subscale was randomly split into two halves and every time a split-half reliability was computed. The process was repeated till we got the maximum possible split-half reliability of 0.89; thus, the obtained two halves had correlations of 0.97 each with the mood reaction scale and of 0.92 and 0.90 with the overall psychological recovery scale. These two halves termed as short version 1 and short version 2 are given in Appendix B. The Cronbach alphas (αs) for these two short versions were 0.81 and 0.80, respectively.

Psychological Recovery and Background Variables

Three background variables education, age and income were correlated with four subscales and overall measures of recovery. These correlations are presented in Table 7.3.

The emerging pattern shows that in general background variables of age and income had no relationship with psychological recovery. Only education had positive relation with mood state and positive orientation subscales and the overall scale, meaning that higher the education of the patients, lower was the positive mood and higher was the positive orientation, the higher was the overall psychological recovery.

Similarly the relative's assessment had positive correlation with education of the patient. The doctor's assessment, interestingly, had significant correlations with all three background variables, that is, the higher the education, the lower the age and income, the higher was doctor's assessment of patient's recovery.

Table 7.4 presents the mean recovery ratings of the patients having different types of health problems. It seems that all the patients show a similar mean pattern for all the measures of recovery, including those of doctor's and relative's. It, however, seems that responses on psychosomatic symptoms were consistently higher and on positive orientation consistently lower than on other two scales. On these other two scales

Table 7.3:

Correlations of background characteristics with measures of psychological recovery, doctor's and relative's assessment

Subscales	Background Characteristics		
	Education	*Age*	*Income*
Illness appraisal	0.19	0.05	0.13
Psychosomatic symptoms	0.08	−0.11	−0.12
Mood state	0.28*	−0.12	0.12
Positive orientation	0.28*	−0.13	0.15
Overall	**0.31***	**−0.09**	**0.13**
Doctor's assessment	0.39*	−0.31*	−0.45*
Relative's assessment	0.29	0.04	0.18

*$p < 0.01$. $n = 80$.

Table 7.4:
Mean psychological recovery of four categories of patients

Subscales	Category of Patients			
	Surgery	*Heart*	*Cancer*	*Orthopaedic*
Illness appraisal	2.66	2.72	2.70	2.78
Psychosomatic symptoms	3.88	3.82	3.40	3.83
Mood state	2.40	2.63	2.33	2.75
Positive orientation	2.26	1.84	2.13	2.33
Overall	**2.62**	**2.68**	**2.51**	**2.82**
Doctor's assessment	2.16	2.82	2.79	3.07
Relative's assessment	2.68	2.72	2.56	2.76

the responses were mostly on the somewhat lower than the mid-point of the scale. The observed frequency distributions of these subscales also did not differ.

Discussion

A measure of psychological recovery of the hospital patients was developed in the present study. The psychometric criteria of selecting items in the scale were response variability, discrimination among the patients' low and high on the overall score, homogeneity of the scale items and sensitivity to tap the change over time. The scale thus can be a useful tool in testing intra-individual changes as response to the hospitalization, as well as, to assess individual and group differences. Another strength of the scale is its comprehensibility; mapping psychological recovery from various standpoints, namely appraisal of illness, psychosomatic symptoms, mood state and positive orientation. The scale is in simple Hindi and can be administered in about 30 minutes. In fact, if time and illness of the patient is a constraint, two shorter versions of the scale are also prepared, each taking not more than 10 minutes. These two short versions can be handy for repeated measurement in pre- and post-conditions.

The scale has internal consistency as was confirmed by consistently high Cronbach alphas. The four different subscales had high correlations with the summated scale. As the need may be, these subscales can be used independently. The scale has discriminant validity as a measure of temporal change. Further work is needed to establish its concurrent and construct validity. The scale obviously has some of the limitations of a verbal measure. Particularly when the patients are preoccupied with the illness and its after-effects (like acute pain or sensory dullness), they cannot clearly appraise their internal state. This scale is, thus, not very useful in the cases of acute and terminal diseases.

Notwithstanding, this psychological recovery scale can be used on a wide range of patients suffering from different chronic diseases. With minor changes in wordings, it can be used in cases of other diseases and disabilities. Again, the scale can be used for non-hospital patients with some changes. There is no restriction of the disease duration for the scale to be used. The only condition is that illness should still have serious implications for the respondents. All those patients who are mentally fit and not under intensive care can complete this scale. The scale is developed on non- and semi-literate individuals coming from rural areas. The idea was that if these scale items can be comprehended by them, it should be easy for the educated sample.

It should be noted that there was no correlation between psychological recovery and the recovery as assessed by the attending doctor. Doctors, it seems, use different criteria to appraise recovery of the patients, the one used by the patient and the other used by their close attendant. That the doctors differ in their judgements from patients and relatives was also found in other studies. For example, in one study of hypertension (Jachuk et al., 1982) it was found that although 100% of the physicians reported their patients have improved following medication, only half of the patients agreed and none of the relatives did. In Indian government hospitals where patients come in contact with the doctors for a very brief period and the interaction is very formal, doctors hardly come to know their patients. Their recovery assessments are based more on the demographic background of the patient, such as age, education and income. It was evident from the findings of this study.

The psychological recovery scale can be used for a variety of purposes in psychological research. The scale may be complementary to various measures of medical recovery. This information could be useful in deciding the further course of treatment, and in also determining the extent to which the patient can take self-care and can follow treatment regimen. It could be used for diagnostic purpose. To assess the mental health of the patients in terms of neurotic anxiety, depression, psychosomatic symptoms, etc., the scale items selectively interpreted could be informative of social and emotional adjustment of the patients. Such information is as important as hard medical data in predicting completing recovery of the patients (Taylor, 2006).

After a three-decade-long research in this field, we still do not know what pattern psychological recovery follows. Silver and Wortman (1980) raised this issue and concluded that there are no clear findings. Radley (1994) made similar observations more recently. Recovery is influenced by a vast array of factors, such as the nature and severity of the disease, dispositions of the patients, coping strategies employed, and support network. These factors probably also determine what is the nature of the recovery curve. Is it linear, cyclic, asymptotic or with many spikes? Depending on only such understanding of psychological recovery, a future course of action can be planned. More important in this context is that in all diagnostic and treatment-related decisions, patient's perspective acquires significance in the recent times, hereto not considered important in the medical model of health care. The present measure can be an important tool to examine mind-body interaction.

The measure developed here is already employed in two doctoral studies (Kohli, 1995; Singh, 1998). In both of these studies, psychological recovery scale was used to study the role of cultural beliefs in augmenting psychological recovery. These studies not only provided evidences that the scale is functional but also exhibited the facilitating role of cultural beliefs, particularly of metaphysical beliefs in coping with chronic diseases.

Appendix A: Psychological Recovery Scale

Section A: Illness Appraisal

We would be asking you few questions related to your health. We all differ in the way we feel and react when we fall sick. Here, we are interested in knowing how do you view your own illness; how do you feel and react to it?

We would ask you questions, like 'how much improvement you see in your health more recently?' What would you say less or more? You can tell us how much more or much less improvement? In the same way, you will be required to answer each question stated below by checking one of the five categories: very less (1), less (2), somewhat (3), much (4) and very much (5).

	Very Much	Much	Somewhat	Less	Very Less
	1	2	3	4	5
In your assessment, how sick are you?	1	2	3	4	5
In comparison to your earlier assessment, how sick are you now?	1	2	3	4	5
In comparison to other patients with similar problem, how sick are you?	1	2	3	4	5
How fast is your recovery in comparison to other hospital patients?	1	2	3	4	5
To what extent your recovery is within your control?	1	2	3	4	5
How worried are you about your relapse?	1	2	3	4	5
How much hopeful are you that the treatment will be effective?	1	2	3	4	5
How satisfied are you with your treatment?	1	2	3	4	5
How serious you think your sickness is?	1	2	3	4	5
*How much keen are you to find out, what you can do to recover?	1	2	3	4	5
How much worried you are about what future has in store for you?	1	2	3	4	5
How feasible is it for you to take care of your health?	1	2	3	4	5

(Continued)

(Continued)

	Very Much	Much	Somewhat	Less	Very Less
	1	2	3	4	5
*How much effort are you making to recover?	1	2	3	4	5
How much informed are you about your treatment?	1	2	3	4	5

Section B: Psychosomatic Symptoms

During sickness some other symptoms may also start showing up, like increased blood pressure. Please think of any such changes you have noticed in you after falling sick (or in the last month). Like, you may specify, 'how much has your blood pressure increased or decreased or remained the same during that period'. Use the scale given below to indicate your response.

	Decreased	Somewhat Decreased	Same	Somewhat Increased	Increased
	5	4	3	2	1
Loss of appetite	5	4	3	2	1
Difficulty in Breathing	5	4	3	2	1
Loss of sleep	5	4	3	2	1
Bodily weakness	5	4	3	2	1
*Palpitation of Heart	5	4	3	2	1
*Irritability	5	4	3	2	1
Fatigue	5	4	3	2	1
Indigestion	5	4	3	2	1

Section C: Mood State

During sickness some changes in behaviour and thinking are natural. Here you will be asked about such changes in yourself. Keeping in mind your personal experiences of going through this sickness, please tell us how often in a day you feel/think as stated below. Please respond to each statement given below by checking one of the answers—always, often, sometimes, occasionally or never.

	Never	At Times	Sometimes	Often	Always
	5	4	3	2	1
Irritation at the slightest pretext	5	4	3	2	1
Intolerance for noise	5	4	3	2	1
Lack of concentration	5	4	3	2	1
Memory lapse	5	4	3	2	1
Anger without provocation	5	4	3	2	1
Desire to keep others happy	5	4	3	2	1
*Feel like telling others about my problems	5	4	3	2	1
Feel like crying	5	4	3	2	1
Restlessness	5	4	3	2	1
Desire to avoid people	5	4	3	2	1
Nothing feels good	5	4	3	2	1
Difficulty in taking decisions	5	4	3	2	1
Mental tension	5	4	3	2	1
Feel hurt by others' comments	5	4	3	2	1
Sympathy for other patients	5	4	3	2	1
Apprehensive	5	4	3	2	1
*Thoughts of others' suffering	5	4	3	2	1
Fear of worse happenings	5	4	3	2	1
Fear of desertion by own people	5	4	3	2	1
Fear of loneliness	5	4	3	2	1
Feeling that everything will be fine eventually	5	4	3	2	1
Pessimistic thoughts	5	4	3	2	1
Anxiety about the future	5	4	3	2	1
Desire to laugh and joke	5	4	3	2	1
Feeling that stars are on my side	5	4	3	2	1
Feeling that things are going my way	5	4	3	2	1

Section D: Positive Orientation

Please indicate to what extent do you agree with the statements given below.

	Very Much	Much	Somewhat	Less	Very Less
	5	4	3	2	1
Good days always follow bad days	5	4	3	2	1
Whatever God does, does for our good	5	4	3	2	1
Suffering makes people wiser	5	4	3	2	1
Future days will be good	5	4	3	2	1
If people try they can sail through any crisis	5	4	3	2	1
Every problem has a solution	5	4	3	2	1
Problems never come alone, they follow one another*	5	4	3	2	1
One can change one's destiny	5	4	3	2	1

*These items in the scale were deleted from the final version.

Appendix B: Psychological Recovery Scale (Shorter Version 1)

Instructions

During sickness some changes in behaviour and thinking are natural. Here, you will be asked about such changes in yourself. Keeping in mind your personal experiences of going through this sickness, please tell us how often in a day you feel/think as stated below. Please respond to each statement given below by checking one of the answers—always, often, sometimes, occasionally or never.

	Never	Occasionally	Sometimes	Often	Always
	5	4	3	2	1
2. Intolerance for noise	5	4	3	2	1
3. Lack of concentration	5	4	3	2	1
4. Memory lapses	5	4	3	2	1
8. Feel like crying	5	4	3	2	1
11. Nothing feels good	5	4	3	2	1
12. Difficulty in taking decisions	5	4	3	2	1
14. Feel hurt by others' comments	5	4	3	2	1
15. Sympathy for other patients	5	4	3	2	1
18. Fear of worse happenings	5	4	3	2	1
20. Fear of loneliness	5	4	3	2	1
24. Desire to laugh and joke	5	4	3	2	1
26. Feel that things are going my way	5	4	3	2	1

The remaining 12 items of Scale 3 constitute Shorter Version 2 of Psychological Recovery Scale.

8

Measures of Perception of Hospital Environment and Affective Reactions

People are generally admitted to hospitals when an illness reaches an advanced stage of severity, disrupting normal life activities, when all other modes of treatment fail and when specialized treatment and close monitoring becomes essential. People generally fear and avoid hospitalization as long as they can. The general stereotype of hospitals is that of a place where people suffer and die. Hospitalization uproots the patients from their familiar surroundings, strips them off their social roles and identity, and renders their usual style of functioning ineffective. Patients feel trapped in an alien, impersonal environment and are intimidated by rigid hospital schedules, rules and regulation. Hospital imposes many restrictions on the activities of its inmates, who are expected to conform to certain normative pattern of behaviour. They are guided and monitored by doctors, nurses and ancillary staff of the hospital. Hospital thus creates an environment for the patient, which is very different from their familiar home environment (Reuben and Omorilewa, 1991). Hospitalization itself is, thus, a major cause of stress for the patients. One's recovery from the disease is much dependent on how he or she perceives hospital environment, adapts to its demands, and copes with the anxieties and threat it causes.

The stresses related to hospitalization may be diverse; some may be related to patients' familial and financial conditions, others may be related to hospital staff and physical environment, and still others are related to their disease conditions, which impinge on patients' recovery from the disease. Equally important is patients' own perception of the hospital environment, which plays a crucial role in their response to their health condition and mobilizing internal resources to get well. To be precise, it is argued and empirically examined in this paper that there are close linkages between perceived hospital environment and patients' emotive reactions, which implicate their recovery process.

It has been known since ages that patients' recovery from a disease condition greatly depends on the psychosocio-physical environment in which they get treatment. In the Indian tradition, Ayurvedic physicians stressed proper care, diet, hygiene and secured environment as essential requisites for holistic recovery from a disease (Raina, 1990). The ancient Roman physician Galen recognized the crucial role of healing environment in recovery of the patients (Pearcy, 1985). Florence Nightingale was also famed for her focus on sanitation and other aspects of the environment that contribute to the health and healing of the patients. Stichler (2001), in her review of related research, reports that patients experience positive outcomes when the environment incorporates natural light, elements of nature, peaceful colours, soothing sounds, pleasant views and an overall pleasing aesthetic essence. Recent research suggests that the immune system can be enhanced or suppressed by external stimuli and that the brain reacts to external stimuli at an unconscious level (Malkin, 2003). The physiological effect of stress negatively affects patients' ability to heal. Creating physical environments that support families' and patients' psychological well-being, by contrast, can produce a positive impact on therapeutic outcomes, reduce stressors and improve staff performance and morale (Lusk and Lash, 2005).

Many studies have shown that in the United States, visit to a hospital is often considered to be stressful by patients and their family members. Long-term hospitalization is not only a drain on patients' financial and social resources, but also it makes patients vulnerable to psychological stresses, consequently lowering their immunity and making them susceptible to hospital-acquired infections. In fact, hospital-acquired infections are among the leading causes of death in the United States, killing more Americans than AIDS, breast cancer and automobile accidents (Institute of Medicine, 2004). According to WHO (2010), of every 100 hospitalized patients at any given time, seven in developed and 10 in developing countries will acquire at least one health care–associated infection. The frustration level of both patients and clinicians has probably never been higher and is now on the rise. Though a majority of patients still get well as a result of hospitalization, hospitals remind of all negative imageries and is held as a place to be avoided (Smith and Crawford, 2004).

The hospital as an organization has become increasingly complex in today's world. Because of the diversity of treatment needs, many different kinds of skills and expertise are required in hospitals. There are specialized departments and medical professionals. A hospital has to constantly deal with all kinds of emergencies to save lives. There are conflicts of interest between administrative, medical and paramedical staff. As an open system, hospitals exist within a historical and socio-political context. They are very much affected by the prevailing cultural ethos and belief system of the patients and their families. Given the scarcity of resources and manpower, and the political patronage, Indian hospitals work under too many constraints. The physical environment of most government hospitals is far from satisfactory. There is foul odour, filth, noise, poor sanitation and unrestricted flow of people. The resource-starved and poorly managed hospitals are hardly able to provide supposedly free services to all those who turn up.

Hospitals in India have an urban bias. In 1998, there were 137,006 sub-centres, 23,179 primary health centres and 2,913 community health centres in India. There were 665,639 hospital beds or 6.9 hospital beds per 10,000 persons. According to Health Information of India (1998), out of the total number of 7,765 government hospitals, 6,131 (nearly 79%) are located in cities, where doctors and nurses are educated in the western medicinal system. The lifestyle, language and urban culture of the medical staff do not instil confidence and assurance in the patients, who (in government hospitals particularly) primarily come from the rural and lower socio-economic strata of the society (Dalal, 2013; Latha and Shankar, 2011). The cultural and status differentials between the patients and the doctors often result in patients submitting to the authority of their doctors. Patients' hopes and despairs are contingent on the pleasures and displeasures of their attending doctors, who are seen as almighty saviours. To a hapless patient, who is caught in the cobweb of complex hospital system, even the lower down paramedical staff appears too invincible to be displeased. In such an environment, the patients have to forgo personal control over their lives; all major decisions about them being taken by those who are strangers to them. The hospital ethos, thus, has no congruity with the patients' life in the outside world.

Patient's perception of health-care system is still ignored by the health-care managers in the developing countries. Most of these studies are conducted by medical personnel, funded by Indian Council of Medical Research or similar state agencies. These studies have a medical bias, which is evident in their findings. Taking factors related to patient satisfaction, such as quality of clinical services provided, availability of medicine, behaviour of doctors and other health staff, cost of the services, hospital infrastructure, physical comfort, emotional support and respect for patient preferences, Sodani and Sharma (2011) conducted a study in the hospitals of Madhya Pradesh. They found that though hospitals were overcrowded, patients who were primarily from rural areas were satisfied with many aspects of hospital environment. Similar findings were obtained by Singh (2011) in his study of government hospitals in Haryana. Shah (2010), in a study of district hospitals in Kolkata, observed that infrastructure of government hospitals is very inadequate to handle a large number of patients and thus are unable to provide services to all. Patients have to come 2–3 times and wait for hours to meet the doctor. Another study showed that in India 80% of the health-care expenses are borne by the users, 90% of which are by the poor people (Krishnakumar, 2004).

On hospitalization, patients' discomfort is aggravated by the depersonalized treatment they receive. In the hospital, a patient is just a number, or a case, or a body to be medicated or operated upon. The patients are expected to remain passive, cooperative and conforming to the treatment procedure. Such role expectations from the patients are universal, but more apt in Indian set-up due to illiteracy, and poverty of the majority of patients, and heavy role demands on medical staff. In the perennially overcrowded Indian hospitals, the doctors have to attend a long array of in-door and out-door patients, besides serving as teachers and administrators. Any attempt by doctors to be personal in their approach result in patients putting more demands on doctor's time and services, and the possibility of leaving many patients unattended. For the hospital staff, depersonalization may serve as a coping strategy who must deal with death and suffering on a daily basis.

Such depersonalization also emanates from bureaucracy and routinization of treatment procedures of allopathic system of medicine

(Goffman, 1961). Besides, constantly changing duties of junior doctors and nursing staff, and shifting of the patients from one ward to another do not allow any personal relationship to develop. The era of super-specialization in the medical system is further enhancing the sense of depersonalization. Mostly these specialists who take treatment-related decisions are strangers to the patients. The specialists come in contact with the patients for a short time and deal with a very specific aspect of their problem. Depersonalization of patients does not fit within the dominant Indian cultural ethos, where most of the social and professional interactions are personalized (Kakar and Kakar, 2007). People tend to feel very anxious in an impersonal situation.

Another important factor that shapes hospital environment is doctor–patient communication. An observation commonly shared by patients is that their doctors have neither time nor inclination to inform them about the diagnosis and treatment course. In a study conducted in four government hospitals of Delhi, Pathak (1979) found that about 50% of the patients reported rude behaviour of hospital staff as the major difficulty experienced during hospitalization. Doctors do not find it necessary to provide correct information about patients' illness or about the treatment procedures. Because of the status differential, patients are generally afraid of asking questions to their doctors and are generally ill-informed about their illness. As found by Ford and colleagues (1996), cancer patients in a London teaching hospital were often asked closed than open-ended questions by the clinicians. Patients asked even fewer questions and were given little scope to initiate any discussion. During their rounds, doctors refer patients in terms of cases, disease and other physical conditions. They discuss among themselves in technical jargons, being totally oblivious of the presence of the patient who is the focus of all discussions. Language becomes barrier in doctor–patient communication, as often doctors do not understand local dialect. Even when the information is provided, it is often vague and incomprehensible, which further enhances the patients' anxiety. In one study of surgical patients, Dalal and Singh (1992) found that 60% of the patients in the government hospitals did not have even the basic information about the kind of surgery they were undergoing. Banerjee and Sanyal (2012) reported that patients' communication with their doctor is passive and one-sided and in 40% of the cases they do not trust their doctor. Doctors also seem to underestimate patients' ability to comprehend information about their diagnosis and treatment.

The doctors, in essence, are educated to focus on curative or biological aspects of the disease. Psychosocial aspects of the disease are either ignored or superficially dealt with. The doctors do not receive any formal training to deal with anxieties, fears and other emotional crises of the patients. This further mars the doctor–patient communication. Carstairs and Kapur (1976) observed that the Indian patients primarily look for symptom relief and alleviation of anxiety. Since the doctors are unable to attend patients' anxiety, most of the times, the patients are dissatisfied with their communication with the doctors.

Another barrier in doctor–patient communication is divergent beliefs about the illness, its meaning, causes and recovery process. Patients frequently attribute their illness to metaphysical factors and resort to traditional health practices. While visiting a hospital, patients are not usually so much interested in technical details of their disease. Their interest is in knowing about the correct diagnosis, seriousness of the disease, causes of the disease and side effects of the medication. The information they receive from the doctors is usually about the organic malfunctioning and the treatment regimen (Dalal, 2013). Patients are very much inhibited to discuss with the doctor their fears and anxieties. In fact, major sources of information for most of the patients are other patients, their visitors and lower order paramedical staff. Such faulty doctor–patient communication often results in imprecise diagnosis and low compliance.

Patients' Coping Reactions

The manner in which patients react to hospitalization largely depends on those specific features of the environment, which affect the patients most. Some people associate hospitals with dreadful things such as pain and death; others are more disturbed by the dehumanizing process of treatment. Some patients do not like the disruptiveness of hospital stay, the extreme dependency and loss of control. Some patients react more to complex, confusing, chaotic hospital environment, and to the noise, crowd and repulsive odour. There are still other people who are most disturbed by the lack or ambiguity of information. Such variation in the patients' coping reaction would also depend on demographic background—age, gender, education, income, etc.

Taylor (1979) identified that the characteristic responses of patients to their loss of control in the hospital setting are that of anger, helplessness, depression, anxiety and withdrawal. These negative feelings in a way exacerbate the perception of hospital environment and the patients get into a vicious cycle. It may be noted that all the affective reactions do not have negative consequences. For example, Janis and Rodin (1979) found that anticipatory fear in surgical patients give rise to a rehearsal mechanism called 'work of worrying'. Work of worrying with adequate information mentally prepares patients to face the adverse consequences in the face of uncontrollable life events. In her review of oncology research in India, Malhotra (2008) has noted some of the reactions that patients manifest in such a set-up.

The narratives as recounted by hospital patients in western societies reveal feelings of helplessness, of losing control, of victimization and shame (Kleinman, 1986; Sahin et al., 2007). In Indian situation, acceptance than reactance is found to be the characteristic response. People frequently attribute their illness to supernatural causes. Theory of Karma provides the causal explanations for all happenings in life, including health problems (Paranjpe, 1984, 1998). As a part of Karma theory, people believe in *prarabdh*, which means that once a crisis starts unfolding itself it will complete its course and no efforts can wish it away. People in crisis thus try to transcend the obnoxious situation, or derive some positive meaning in their suffering. These patients are expected to be less affected by the hospital environment and manifest less extreme affective reactions.

Often it is difficult to isolate those coping responses, which are specific to the hospitalization and not to the severity of disease they suffer from. The coping reactions would also vary with illness episodes and in different phases of hospitalization. Though patients make some predictable responses to their hospitalization, or to some aspects of hospital environment, such emotions are often general reactions to their predicament. This study, thus, examined the common pattern of coping reactions which patients suffering from different diseases show as reaction to their hospitalization.

To sum up, this study had three major objectives:

1. To develop a Perceived Hospital Environment Scale and a Coping with Hospitalization Scale for patients in Indian hospitals.

2. To examine how hospital patients differ on these two measures along demographic variables.
3. To map relation between Perceived Hospital Environment and Coping with Hospitalization.

Method

Sample of the Hospital Patients

The patients were randomly selected from the general wards of the Swaroop Rani Hospital, Allahabad. This is the largest government hospital where the treatment is free of charge. In all, 122 patients were interviewed. Of these, 86 were males and 34 were females, their age ranging between 25 and 55 years, average age being 38 years. These patients were in hospital for at least one week, primarily suffering from chronic abdominal ($n = 32$), respiratory ($n = 18$), orthopaedic ($n = 43$) and miscellaneous ($n = 29$) health problems. There were no patients whose disease was acute or life threatening. Total 102 of these patients were admitted in the hospital for the first time, for the rest it was a case of readmission.

These patients were from the same population as taken in the earlier studies. They were predominantly from the rural background and had travelled long distances to get treatment. Each patient was accompanied by some close relative. The modal education of this sample was of primary level, 70% female and 35% male had no formal education. About 80% of the patients came from lower and lower middle class and their monthly family income was below ₹2,500.

Operationalization of Two Measures

In this exploratory study, two separate measures were prepared: one for the perception of hospital environment and the other for mapping patients' affective reactions. Perceived hospital environment was operationalized as patients' understanding and response to physical setting, disease threat and security, communication with hospital staff, restrictions and sense of well-being. These features of patient's reactions were culled out from existing literatures on hospitalization of physical and psychiatric patients. Studies dealing with the patients who were terminally sick were avoided.

For developing a measure of coping responses of the patients, coping was conceptualized in a broader sense to include both affective and cognitive responses. Behavioural responses were mostly not included in this scale and as these are contingent of many other considerations. Affective reactions included in the study were similar to those taken in other studies, like feeling sadness, anger, depression, rejection, etc. The cognitive responses were intended to map their thinking pattern in response to environmental stresses. The idea was to include those response patterns, which are typical of Indian patients in government hospitals.

Interview Schedule

The interview schedule developed for the hospital patients had three sections. Section 1 dealt with the general background, including demographic and illness background of the patients.

Section 2 was a measure of Perceived Hospital Environment. There were 40 Likert-type statements, which were prepared on the basis of open-ended interviews with 15 patients. These statements were further revised and selected on the basis of a pilot study on 10 patients and in consultation with other colleagues in the Psychology Department. The statements that were retained covered diverse aspects of organizational environment, specifically those which are relevant to the prevailing environment in Indian hospitals. The aggregate score on this measure would be indicative of favourable–unfavourable environment.

Section 3 was yet another measure, prepared to tap the affective reactions of the patients in Indian hospitals. These affective reactions were indicative of the way patients respond to their hospitalization. There were 36 items in this measure, each from one of the following six categories: anger, anxiety, depression, helplessness, disengagement and rationalization. All these items were rated by the patients along a 5-point rating scale, on which 1 implied rarely and 5 implied always felt that way. The preliminary scale was revised and refined on the basis of the data of the same pilot study ($n = 10$) as mentioned earlier.

The final form of these two scales are given in Appendices A and B.

Patients in the study were also asked how much physical pain they were experiencing these days on a 5-point scale.

Data Collection

The interviews with the patients were conducted in the hospital premises with the permission of the attending doctor, patients and their attendants. The patients were informed about the purpose of the study and an appointment was sought. The patients were ensured complete confidentiality and were told that these interview data will be used only for the purpose of research. During interviews in few cases, patients' family members were present.

In most of the cases, the interview took about 30–50 minutes. Except in three cases where the patients wanted a break, all other interviews were completed in one session. In the beginning, the general information about the patients' background and about their illness was sought.

Before administering the hospital environment and affective reaction measures, patients were made familiar with the 5-point scales. They were given a pictorial scale in which the blocks of squares uniformly increased in size. The smallest block was identified as 1 and the largest as 5, and so on. Each statement was read to the patients and their responses were recorded. The patients were assured that there were no right or wrong answers. The interviews were conducted by a research staff member who had doctoral degree in psychology and was experienced in this type of research.

Results

Perceived Hospital Environment Scale

This scale had 40 items and on the basis of mean, SD and item-total correlations, all the items were retained. These items were then subjected to varimax factor rotation. Six factors whose Eigen values were above 0.85 were retained. These factors taken together predicted 48% of the total variance. Highest (sometimes close second) factor loadings

Table 8.1:
Perceived hospital environment scale

Dimension	No. of Items	Item	M	SD	Cronbach α
Physical environment	6	3, 4, 8, 11, 32, 37	3.00	0.73	0.59
Treatment facility	7	12, 14, 15, 16, 22, 35, 38	3.42	0.47	0.39
Doctor–patient communication	7	6, 17, 18, 19, 23, 28, 29	3.14	0.61	0.58
Social environment	7	1, 7, 9, 13, 20, 26, 39	3.09	0.45	0.09
Perceived control	7	5, 24, 25, 27, 30, 33, 34	2.22	0.53	0.46
Sense of security	6	2, 10, 21, 31, 36, 40	3.16	0.59	0.65
Overall	40		3.0	0.36	0.66

Note: Higher score implies more positive perception.

were the criteria to categorize items along these six factors. Table 8.1 presents summary statistics of this scale.

The first column in Table 8.1 shows the nomenclature of six dimensions (factors) of the scale. The items within these dimensions ranged from 6 to 7. The item numbers as mentioned in the table are the same as in Appendix A. The mean and SD of these dimensions are within normal range; however, Cronbach αs for treatment facility and social environment were low, and therefore need to be interpreted with some caution. The overall alpha (0.66) is high, which suggests that taken as a whole the scale has high internal consistency.

The six dimensions represented different sets of items. The first dimension of *physical environment* includes crowding, noise and hygiene conditions in the hospital. *Treatment conditions* refer to whether or not patients think that they stand good chances of getting well here. *Doctor–patient communication* is indicative of how well patients are informed about their disease and treatment, and how free they feel in making queries. The *social environment* refers to patient's social interaction and support from other patients and hospital staff. *Perceived control* is the sense of freedom/control, which a patient has in the hospital setting. The last dimension is named as *sense of security*, meaning whether a patient finds hospital environment assuring or fear arousing. Scoring for all these dimensions were in positive direction, such that higher scores implied positive perception of hospital environment.

Further analysis revealed that the nature of illness did not significantly influence the perception of hospital environment along any

Table 8.2:
Gender differences in the perception of hospital environment

Dimension	Male (n = 88)	Female (n = 34)	t-test
1. Physical environment	3.10	2.75	2.46*
2. Treatment conditions	3.40	3.47	−0.73
3. Doctor–patient communication	3.20	2.98	1.77
4. Social environment	3.14	2.97	1.94*
5. Perceived control	2.25	2.16	0.91
6. Sense of security	3.36	2.62	4.86**

*$p < 0.05$; **$p < 0.01$.

of the dimension. Also, the first timer or multiple timers did not matter. Gender differences in the perception of hospital environment were observed, which are presented in Table 8.2. It was found that on the hospital dimensions of physical environment and sense of security male patients perceived hospital environment more positive than the female patients. On other dimensions, there was no gender difference.

Measure of Coping with Hospital Stresses

The second measure in the questionnaire pertaining to responses to stressful hospital environment was also subjected to factor analysis. The factors yielded were very large in number (14), accounting for only 52% of the total variance. This was therefore abandoned. To categorize the items, consequently, judges' ratings were resorted to. The items were divided along two dimensions: affective state and thinking state. The items related to the affective state of the patients were put into the categories of anger, anxiety, depression and helplessness. There were three items in each subcategory. The thought-related items were categorized as acceptance, transcendence, positive orientation, recovery orientation and pain-obsession. The number of items in these categories varied from three to six. Mean, SD and Cronbach αs for these sub-measures are given in Table 8.3. Cronbach αs for the sub-measure of pain-obsession was quite low and was dropped from the scale. To improve Cronbach α of acceptance sub-measure, an item having low item-total correlation was deleted. The final measure thus had only 32 items (see Appendix B).

It is quite likely that patients' reactions may be contingent on the nature of their illness and duration of hospitalization. There may be gender differences. Mean comparisons were tested by computing F and t-tests. It was found that duration of hospitalization was not a significant variable as far as patients' coping responses were concerned. Mean comparisons for the nature of illness and gender differences are reported in Table 8.4.

Table 8.3:
Coping responses to hospitalization

Dimension	Items	Mean	SD	Cronbach α
Affective	**12**	**2.08**	**0.48**	**0.63**
Anger	3	1.63	0.57	0.53
Anxiety	3	1.75	0.61	0.37
Depression	3	2.62	0.80	0.53
Helplessness	3	2.32	0.77	0.55
Cognitive	**21**	**2.47**	**0.33**	**0.58**
Acceptance	5	2.80	0.46	0.25
Transcendence	6	2.47	0.50	0.56
Positive orientation	4	2.35	0.62	0.50
Recovery cognitions	6	2.29	0.45	0.48

Table 8.4:
Coping responses across nature of health problem and gender

	Health Problem				Gender		
Dimension	Abdominal $n = 32$	Orthopaedic $n = 43$	Other $n = 45$	F $(2, 117)$	M $n = 88$	F $n = 34$	t-test
Affective	**3.02**	**2.79**	**3.00**	**3.04***	**2.00**	**2.30**	**3.16**
Anger	3.36	3.43	3.34	0.34	1.55	1.85	2.70*
Anxiety	3.25	3.16	3.33	0.85	1.66	2.00	2.87*
Depression	2.56	2.12	2.51	3.85*	2.55	2.81	1.60
Helplessness	2.89	2.43	2.80	4.12*	2.25	2.52	1.77
Cognitive	**2.67**	**2.45**	**2.51**	**4.28****	**2.54**	**2.31**	**–3.58****
Acceptance	2.36	2.06	2.22	4.01*	2.86	2.64	–2.50**
Transcendence	2.69	2.41	2.55	3.03*	2.55	2.38	–2.65**
Positive orientation	2.85	2.63	2.57	2.15	2.44	2.19	–2.96**
Recovery cognitions	2.79	2.70	2.67	0.62	2.32	2.21	–1.27

Note: All values are in positive direction, that is, greater score implies more positive state.
*$p < 0.05$; **$p < 0.01$.

The patients were classified into three categories: abdominal, orthopaedic and other (or miscellaneous). F test and further mean comparison showed that orthopaedic patients were less depressed and helpless in comparison to abdominal and other patients. In general, orthopaedic patients were less emotionally disturbed, even though they were less accepting of their misery and were less engaged in transcendence (spiritual thinking). Patients of three categories showed similar reactions along other sub-measures.

As far as gender differences were concerned, female than male patients showed more anger and anxiety, and in general more emotional reaction. On cognitive dimension, female patients showed more acceptance, transcendence and positive orientation than the male patients.

Table 8.5 shows the correlations of hospital environment measures with coping responses of the patients. A perusal of these correlations suggest that, overall, there is a significant positive relationship between affective coping responses and hospital environment. That is, the more favourable perception of hospital environment they have the more positive affective state they exhibit. In particular, sense of security in hospital was highly correlated with positive emotional state. Congenial doctor–patient relationship, social environment and sense of security

Table 8.5:
Correlations between perceived hospital environment and coping responses

| Coping Dimension | Hospital Environment (Dimensions) | | | | | | |
	1	*2*	*3*	*4*	*5*	*6*	*Overall*
Affective	28*	10	33**	28	16	56**	48**
Anger	20	–03	12	12	–13	37**	19
Anxiety	24*	20	29**	05	10	42**	37**
Depression	17	11	17	20	21	38	35
Helplessness	18	–01	32**	35**	20	39**	40**
Cognitive	**–05**	**04**	**07**	**–09**	**13**	**02**	**03**
Acceptance	–07	06	15	–12	17	05	07
Transcendence	–02	–07	02	–10	13	03	01
Positive orientation	–12	–14	–07	–04	–06	–08	–14
Recovery thoughts	06	25*	09	02	16	05	15

$^*p < 0.05$; $^{**}p < 0.01$.

were associated with less helplessness. Perceived hospital environment did not correlate with cognitive dimension of the coping responses, except in the case of treatment facility and recovery orientation.

Discussion

The present study had twin goals. One, to develop measures of hospital stress and that of coping responses of the patients, and two, to examine relationship between hospital stress and coping responses. Keeping in view that little work is done in this area of taking patients' perspective, the findings of the present study throw useful light on the way patients in Indian hospitals perceive their environment. The prevailing socio-cultural and physical environment of Indian hospitals sets them apart from their western counterparts, notwithstanding the fact that they are modelled on western medical system.

The perceived hospital environment measure covered physical, social, personal and medical aspects, providing an overall patient evaluation of a government hospital. The orthogonal axis-rotation yielded neat six dimensions with items uniformly distributed. The statistical data further revealed that mean and SD of these sub-measures were in the normal range and Cronbach α is consistently high, except for the sub-measure of 'treatment facilities'. The overall Cronbach α (0.66) was on the higher side. At present, the test has content and factor-analytic validity; its criterion validity could not be established in the absence of another known India measure.

It was further observed that earlier exposure to hospital environment did not affect patients' present evaluation, nor did the nature of their physical health problem. The demographic background also did not change the response pattern, except some gender differences. In that the male patients perceived hospital environment more positively in terms of physical environment and sense of security than the female patients. A notable feature of this measure is that it can be administered on the whole range of population, including rural and illiterate on whom this measure was developed. Though developed for the government hospitals, this measure should be useful in mapping perceived environment of the non-government hospitals as well.

The range and nature of hospital environment dimensions derived from the factor analysis substantiate the point that there is underlying similarity in patients' perceptions in different cultural settings. In many western studies (e.g. Nienke, 2012) measures of perceived hospital environment are inclusive of these dimensions.

Despite the fact that response dimensions are the same, there is a qualitative difference in perception of the patients in Indian hospitals. As Pathak (1979) noted, unfriendly behaviour of hospital staff was reported by more than 51% of the patients as a major difficulty during hospitalization. Due to overcrowding and inadequate staffing, medical needs of the patients are barely attended to, not to speak of the psychological needs that go largely unnoticed. Understandably, as Pathak found, 55% of the patients are admitted in the hospital for acute symptoms and as many as 63% of them leave the hospital after symptomatic relief. These data are revealing of the free treatment facilities in the government hospitals, which are mostly used by the poor section of the society. These people are less demanding and have low expectations of proper hospital care (Ramani et al., 2008). This possibly explains why on the hospital environment measures, the mean scores are above the mid-point of the scale.

Developing a measure of coping responses of hospital patient was another objective of this study. The two broad dimensions along which all responses were classified are affective and cognitive dimensions. The affective categories were the same as taken in earlier studies (see Taylor et al., 1979; Silver and Wortman, 1980). The cognitive categories are made relevant to the Indian cultural belief system. The mean and SD of these response categories are within the normal range. The Cronbach αs were also above the acceptable level, except for two categories: anxiety and acceptance. The items within these two categories were more diverse, reducing the homogeneity of these two sub-measures. Given the transitory nature of coping responses in a crisis situation (Wortman, 1983), such measures always had problems of standardization. Despite some problems, the present measures of coping responses can be a useful tool for various practical considerations to augment the recovery of the hospital patients.

The behavioural coping responses, which were in the guise of cognitive responses of the patients, showed that in a restrictive hospital environment, patients' freedom to act is severely curtailed. Their behavioural responses of strolling, sleeping, resting, reading and socializing with visitors indicate that the patients were letting the time 'pass'. There were very few responses of information-seeking, participating in the treatment process, or of dealing with the unpleasant environment. Taylor (1979) explains such patient behaviour in terms of helplessness; patients quickly learn in the hospital setting that they have no role in decision-making about themselves. The total dependency on hospital staff leaves little scope for any initiative. Shumaker and Reizenstein (1981) explain it in terms of availability of fewer coping responses to the patients as there is less energy to expend on coping. A third explanation could be in terms of greater cultural readiness of Indian patients to adjust rather than 'act' upon the given situation. Kohli (1995) found in her study that cancer patients had proneness to restructure their cognitions to align them with the existing reality. Examining one's inner world to find the causes of the suffering is what most of the Indian scriptures call for (Radhakrishnan, 1953).

It is interesting to note that orthopaedic patients showed more anger, depression, helplessness but also more acceptance and transcendence than the other patients. As orthopaedic problems have propensity to prolong, the patients were more mentally drained in their efforts to put up with the consequent movement disability. Again, it was found that male patients showed more anger and anxiety than their female patients, who in turn, were more prone to acceptance, transcendence and positive orientation. It could be that the female patients were more conforming to cultural expectations than the male patients. In any case, these findings are at the best empirical generalizations and only further work can establish stability of these findings.

Another finding that deserves attention is that perceived hospital environment had significant correlations only with affective coping responses, but not with cognitive coping responses. Except one, none of the other correlations were significant in case of cognitive coping measures. When the hospital environment was perceived favourably, patients exhibited more positive affective responses. These correlations clearly establish that affective state of the patients is more susceptible to hospital environment. It is, however, difficult to causally link perception of hospital environment with patients coping responses from this correlational nature of the study. At present, these findings are only empirical generalizations and further work is needed to develop a theoretical construct around these correlations.

Appendix A: Perceived Hospital Environment Scale

Instructions

The purpose of this scale is to know how you perceive the environment of the hospital you are presently admitted in. Please read each statement carefully and rate it on a 5-point scale to indicate how much this statement is true for the hospital you are admitted in. Assign one of the scores given below to indicate your response to each of the statements.

1 = not at all, 2 = somewhat, 3 = often, 4 = most of the time and 5 = always

Your responses would be kept confidential and would be used only for the research purpose.

1. I have made many friends with other patients in the ward.
2. In this place I am scared that I will die any day.
3. There is nauseating odour all round in the ward.
4. Noise level in this place is very high.
5. I feel I have no control over my life here.
6. Doctors and nurses give me a smile whenever they pass my bed.
7. I enjoy seeing so many people visiting me from my family.
8. The bed I am sleeping on is not very comfortable.
9. In this ward I feel we all patients are like one family.
10. I feel confident that I have come to the right place for treatment.
11. There is lack of cleanliness in this ward.
12. No nursing staff is present in the ward, except at the time of doctor's visit.
13. My friends in the hospital do care and contribute to my recovery.
14. I am getting proper treatment in this hospital.
15. My recovery is monitored properly here.
16. Medical staff does not bother even when I am in acute pain.
17. Doctors carefully hear when I talk to them about my problems.
18. My attending doctor is least bothered whether I am getting well or not.
19. Doctors are very casual when they come on the round.

20. I feel very lonely here.
21. I get bad dreams in the night and keep worrying about my health.
22. Doctors have correctly diagnosed my problem.
23. Medical staff is very indifferent to my welfare.
24. For doctors and nurses I am just a bed number.
25. I am treated like a small child here who is not consulted about the medication.
26. I keep counting days when I will be out of this place.
27. Doctors don't treat me here like a human being.
28. I am scared to ask any question to my doctor.
29. Doctors only talk in medical language and are least bothered to explain anything.
30. Everyone in this ward is scared of being insulted by the medical staff.
31. I am very worried when no family member is around.
32. I only see misery and death all around me.
33. I feel like running away from this place.
34. I am free here to spend my time the way I want.
35. I am not sure if I am given the right medicines.
36. At this place I am confident that I can handle any emergency.
37. I get enough fresh air and light in my ward.
38. In this hospital even the basic amenities are missing.
39. I don't think anyone here understands what I am going through.
40. My life is now in the hands of God.

Appendix B: Coping with Hospital Stresses Scale

Instructions

During hospitalization one may have a number of thoughts and reactions. Below are listed some such thoughts and reactions which often occur to patients during hospitalization. Kindly check how many times each of it had happened with you in last three days. Your responses would be kept confidential.

	Always	Often	Sometimes	Never
1. Being short tempered	1	2	3	4
2. Anxiety over aggravation of disease	1	2	3	4
3. Have frightening dreams	1	2	3	4
4. Feel helpless	1	2	3	4
5. Get irritated at minor issues	1	2	3	4
6. Think of changing the medicine	1	2	3	4
7. The thought of the pains of other patients	1	2	3	4
8. It seems that nothing can be done by me	1	2	3	4
9. The thought that life is perishable	1	2	3	4
10. To leave everything to fate	1	2	3	4
11. The thought of consulting another doctor	1	2	3	4
12. The thought that whatever is bound to happen will happen	1	2	3	4
13. Feeling of despair prevails	1	2	3	4
14. Do not feel like doing anything	1	2	3	4
15. Concentrate in God	1	2	3	4
16. Think of the past good days	1	2	3	4
17. The thought of having the right treatment	1	2	3	4
18. Spend time in religious discourse	1	2	3	4
19. Fear of indulging in fight with someone	1	2	3	4
20. Having pain in every part of the body	1	2	3	4

(Continued)

(Continued)

	Always	Often	Sometimes	Never
21. Anxious to know how much the improvement is	1	2	3	4
22. Feeling of helplessness prevails	1	2	3	4
23. Feel disgusted by other's sympathy	1	2	3	4
24. It seems that the pain will be unbearable	1	2	3	4
25. It appears that the world is a delusion	1	2	3	4
26. Desire to talk about my disease	1	2	3	4
27. Think of what all I will do after getting well	1	2	3	4
28. Try to forget that I am sick	1	2	3	4
29. Think that joys and sorrows are part of life	1	2	3	4
30. Engross myself in music	1	2	3	4
31. Dream that I am absolutely well	1	2	3	4
32. Think what else should be done to get well	1	2	3	4
33. Keep thinking why should I be the one to be diseased	1	2	3	4
34. Try to get more information to gain health	1	2	3	4
35. The thought comes that there is also a power bigger than man	1	2	3	4
36. Sadness prevails	1	2	3	4

Note: These are English versions of the two scales. There are generic versions of the scales and their reliability and validity should be recomputed for a particular population and context of the study to be conducted.

UNIT III

Chronic Diseases, Self and Society

9

A Narrative Approach to Understand Illness Experience*

The purpose of this chapter is to explore the possibility of applying narrative approach to study illness experiences of the people suffering from chronic diseases. Long-term illnesses often disrupt the taken-for-granted flow of everyday life and call for many readjustments at thinking, emotional and behavioural level. In personal narratives of an illness what people tell is not just a story of an illness but also about their own understanding of the disease and about the efforts they have made to recover. In many recent studies (Roussi and Advi, 2008), narrative method is found to be a useful tool to understand the dynamic interaction between culture, people and disease, and between the mind and the body.

Narrative method in the health psychology has come via medical anthropology, which has argued that narrative analysis is specifically suited to address what is morally and emotionally 'at stake' in health practices (Kleinman and Seeman, 2000). The ethno-methodological studies focused on health beliefs that different ethnic groups had; and the socio-religious rituals, customs and practices that were associated with effective management of illnesses. Participants' stories were obtained to draw inferences about the typical health and illness behaviour of different aboriginal communities. The stories in their own right were not considered useful data and were used only as illustrations to make some

* This chapter is written in collaboration with Shubhra Hajela. Dr Shubhra Hajela is a faculty at the Tata Institute of Social Sciences, Hyderabad Campus.

point. The job of an anthropologist used to be to tease out the data from interviews and observations. The contemporary ethnography has come a long way to accept participants' own stories as valid construal of the reality from the patients' perspective and as one way of representing the 'real' world. The rise of social constructionism has given further impetus to the narrative approach. The emphasis now is on making sense of these stories and to develop some systems of interpreting them. This approach has been very useful in studying indigenous health practices and healing traditions. Kleinman (1988) has extensively used this approach to study how indigenous healing in Asian countries, including India, is effective in case of many diseases.

Narrative as a story where people make meaning out of their illness experience is one of the most common ways of using narratives in health research. Examples of using narratives in this manner include narratives of melancholia (Kangas, 2001) narratives of depression (Kokanovic et al., 2013) narratives of endometriosis (Markovic et al., 2008) and older women's cancer narratives (Sinding and Wiernikowski, 2008). Such studies typically believe that people actively search meaning in their own life experiences and come up with idiosyncratic constructions, which gives them some sense of coherence in the world they live. The content of the story thus reveal this personal meaning. Narratives in health research are employed as exploratory devices to study how people interpret their life events and what constitutes 'illness experience'.

Other strands of narrative research focus on form, structure and function of narrative (Edvardsson et al., 2003; Smith and Sparkes, 2011) and on the co-construction of narratives (Antelius, 2009; Davidsen and Reventlow, 2010; Hydén and Antelius, 2011). Sometimes, narrative research focuses on exploring 'big stories' and 'small stories' in a narrative. 'Big stories' refer to research interviews with minimal interviewer interference, a result of which is a typical biographical account of illness. 'Small stories', on the other hand, refers to ongoing conversations and are generally used in an ethnographic study of illness and disease (Stefen, 2005) of daily mundane life. Such approaches have moved beyond analysing the structural properties of narratives to the process of narration. Another way of differentiating between big and small stories is by differentiating between research questions that ask *what the story is about* versus *how and why is the story told in the first place* (Riessman, 2008). Such approaches thus present myriad ways of using narrative as tools to explore illness experiences.

Whatever is the way of using narrative, most narrative researchers position themselves in between and combine approaches to study the form, process and content of the story told. What also these researchers seem to share is the belief that narratives be used primarily because they take into account the personal, existential and sometimes interpersonal aspects of experience. This is precisely one of the reasons why narratives are used widely in health research.

Popularity of narrative research in the area of chronic illness is also because of its therapeutic healing power (Cashin et al., 2013). What stories seem to do for a person narrating his illness experience is *therapeutic storytelling* (White, 2007). Storytelling is itself liberating as it gives person an opportunity to explore self, make meaning out of circumstances, know others and transform one's thinking. It may also help in finding caring communities that share common practices, values and understandings. Frank (1995) argued that there are three types of 'narratives of illness' prevalent in the writings of people facing illness in themselves or in others: restitution, chaos and quest.

Narrative Construction of Illness Experience

Narrative way of thinking focuses on the uniqueness of individuals as storytellers, as existential beings capable of reflecting back on their lives and making sense of it. The propensity to narrate is ingrained in all human beings; even very young children can tell stories about what happened to them. Bruner (1986) went a step further to suggest a genetic proclivity for narrative understanding. Whether narratives have biological basis is not evident, in traditional cultures narrative way of thinking and doing is a way of communal life (Benham, 2007).

Many writers hold the view that storytelling is the basic human impulse to create order and derive meaning of diverse life experiences. Rankin (2002) argued that a storyteller synthesizes heterogeneous elements like characters, events, circumstances into a coherent temporal narrative, which has a beginning, middle and end or closure. It is to this extent that he believed that narratives can be said to create meaning of experiences. A chronic illness often disrupts the regular flow and drill of everyday life and calls in for adjustments at emotional, physical and behavioural level. During such an instance what people narrate about their illness is what it means to them, how it happened, and the efforts they made to regain their health status. This meaning making, inherent in illness narrative, is important to understand how the patients suffer and cope. Research suggests that those who find meaning in their suffering recover much earlier than those who could not. For instance, Park et al. (2010) noted that finding positive meaning in one's cancer not only led to better mental and physical health but also resulted in spiritual well-being and overall life satisfaction.

Antonovsky (1987) suggested that people try to develop a sense of coherence in the face of acute health stressors. A sense of coherence is a general orientation to render the situation comprehensible, manageable and meaningful. It is an effort to sustain feeling of confidence and hope when things are going wrong. The dynamic process of narrating health stories does help in building up this sense of coherence and preserving integrity of one's own self.

It is also maintained that narrative not only brings an order and meaning to life but also provides structure to the every sense of selfhood. In the process of narration, identities are formed, maintained, questioned and revised. To be identified as a particular person, to be the possessor of various attributes (kind, honest, brave) to be an agent ('I did', 'I said', 'I went'), and to be self-referential ('I felt', 'I realized') is accomplished through stories that give an opportunity for self-revelation and self-construction—giving a sense of individuated self with particular attributes. The very process of narrating involves human agency and imagination, which determines what gets included and excluded in the narrative, how events are plotted and what they are supposed to mean. Individuals, while narrating, construct past events and actions in personal narratives for many purposes one of which is to claim identities and sense of being.

This sense of identity again has some motives and may confer some importance and value to the individual. For example, it is believed that narrations are generally influenced by the prevailing social, political and cultural values. Then if in a particular culture, valour is largely held to be a positive attribute; the narrator will more likely portray self as having much valour or succeeding in all life trials through valour. Narratives thus not only portray individual identity but may also construct identities on the basis of values that are generally congruent with the cultural and social values.

In traditional societies, an illness is a social event, which affects a large number of family and community members. Consequently, many people are involved in facilitating patient's recovery from the illness. A long-term illness quite often jeopardizes one's social relations and status, particularly when one is looking for approval and support. One set of motive the narrator may have is to influence other's perceptions, emotions and inferences. Kakar (2003) suggests that illness stories signify patients' desire to restore their place in family and community. They reaffirm patients' sense of belonging and help in finding cultural moorings. Stories are also intended to restore one's sense of harmony with the spiritual world. This is important particularly in case of those who view their illness as a consequence of some moral transgression.

Gergen (1988) approached the need to narrate from the perspective of language as a tool for communication. He believed that language is a derivative of social interchange. As such, narratives perform various social functions. He illustrated that by using different forms of narratives, each of which fulfilled its function according to its nature. For instance, *stability narrative*—a form of narrative that linked events in a manner that the trajectory of the events remained the same—might reflect an implicit message that one is capable of an enduring, has a coherent identity or that one is capable of persistence in love, commitments, values and goals. Similarly, *progressive narrative*—a form of narrative where there has been an improvement in the situation and where advancement is expected—may reflect on the narrator's need to illustrate positive change, control over circumstances, and a reduction in undesirable characters and circumstances. Another form of narrative, the *regressive narrative*, where conditions have deteriorated and further decrements, may be expected may fulfil the need to arouse attention, sympathy and intimacy.

In a similar vein, Baumeister and Newman (1994) suggested three other motives behind interpretive efforts. One, stories are considered to satisfy the need for self-justification by portraying one's actions as consistent with values, norms and expectations and by expressing intentions in a comprehensible and acceptable manner. Two, stories satisfy the need for self-efficacy by encoding the information about how to control the environment. Stories help in regaining a sense of control over environment, as well as on one's own internal state. Lastly, many stories support the narrator's claim to self-worth by portraying himself or herself as a competent and popular person, that his or her poor health is the cause of concern for so many people, and that his or her illness is putting so many things and plans at stake.

Another reason as to why stories are told by people is to understand the need to convey to others how they have endured circumstances and pass on this experiential knowledge to others. This can be understood as one way in which people confront a dilemma closely posed by Max Weber in a lecture given in 1918 in Munich University, the text of which is known as 'Science as a Vocation'. Weber in that lecture using Tolstoy's prophetic words had remarked—'science is meaningless because it gives no answer to our question, the only question important to us, "what shall we do and how shall we live"' (p. 143). Frank (2002) addressing this very basic question said that the local and contingent solutions that people have found to how they should live are expressed as stories. These stories recount past attempted solutions, which have worked and which have not. They present a way to learn from the past. Thus narratives while construing the past also builds up the present and future. Narratives are seen as critical to the ways in which people transfer an understanding of themselves and their lives, past and present, and how their futures might be.

Narratives are also cathartic to the extent that one may find a channel for legitimate expression. To tell a tale may also give fulfilment to the human need to converse, to share. Psychologists have talked about the human need to tell a tale.

Besides the study of motives as revealed in the individual personal experience, some researchers have also studied the institutional aspects of narratives and what motives get served there. Typically these researchers study what shapes the form of narratives. Contemporary narrative researchers (Chase, 2011) view stories as conditioned by social context, discursive resources and communicative circumstances. These circumstances may include group culture, national culture, institutional settings, social–personal–historical settings as well as formal and informal relations. For example, caregivers of patients tell their stories differently to a doctor than to a relative (Wondrock and Taylor, 2008), differently in a doctor's office than in a counsellor's office (Wampold, 2001) and differently in a diary than to their support group. This suggests that narratives are interpersonally dynamic, produced in a social interaction for a specific audience. Such a view highlights the interactional base of the narrative where narrations move beyond the solitary activity of an individual to a collaborative enterprise—a joint product of the speaker and the listener.

Storytelling Sessions: Re-living Participants' Experiences

Narrative approach calls for a major shift in the relationship between the researcher and the researched. It requires the researcher to relegate his or her position of authority and expertise to a decentred position as a 'participant' or co-constructor of the illness narrative, along with the people suffering from illness. In narrative interviews, patients are considered to be 'naïve psychologists' (Raskin, 2002; Kelley, 1992) capable of analysing and interpreting their illness. It requires a major attitudinal shift where construction of the reality of an illness becomes a joint venture in which the interviewer and the patient are equal partners. The whole atmosphere has to be that of trust, openness, sharing and respect.

The procedure that is used with patients to elicit personal stories is what we call free-floating interviews. The patient and the researcher meet in an informal setting, without any role expectations. There is no agenda, no fixed schedule for the interview but only few research questions to guide the proceeding. The important consideration is to build up trust and confidence, so that the patients feel free to share their experiences. The patients are encouraged to freely associate with their experience of falling sick, in the natural conversational mode. They talk about their own understanding of the illness, about its causality and controllability. The important turning point in the course of their illness and recovery are narrated by the patients. The major coping strategies and resources that the patients had are talked about. It is our experience that the patients have a need to talk and once their initial inhibitions are gone, it use to be difficult to wind up the narrative sessions within any stipulated time frame.

The important consideration is to maintain the condition of informality and spontaneity during the interview. To this end, it is advisable not to begin an interview by asking about the background information. It creates a mental set and structure the interview in a formal format. Again, no personal questions are asked until the patient himself or herself begins to open up. The idea is to let the patient take the initiative and the interviewer follow the lead.

While narrating, people rely on 'autobiographical memory' (Rubin, 1986), which can best be understood as reconstructions rather than reproduction of the past events. As people narrate their illness experiences, past events are reconstructed so as to make them congruent with their current understanding; the present is explained with reference to the reconstructed past; and both are used to generate expectations about the future (Gerro, 1994). Undoubtedly people struggle to account for how they came to be in their present position of suffering and what future might now lie ahead of them. Health and illness thus are intricately interwoven in the fabric of one's life and health stories, which quite often cannot be separated from other life stories. Cultural beliefs, family socialization and life experience all get represented in these health stories.

In particular, central to the construction of an intelligible story a narrator must have a goal, an event to be explained, a state to be reached or avoided, an outcome of significance—or more informally, a point to be made. Once a goal is established, it serves to guides the kinds of events that can subsequently figure in the narrative account. The myriad candidates for 'event-hood' are greatly reduced by establishing the endpoint. An intelligible story is one in which selected events serve to make the goal more or less probable, accessible, important or vivid. Much of this process is not consciously determined but naturally occurs as one proceeds to recount illness experiences.

Again the motive to narrate and the content narrated are guided largely by how institutional selves are created and how institutional boundaries are maintained (Holstein and Gubrium, 2000). It is this institutional context that will shape the beginning of the story, events and characters included in the story and derive morals and learning. It is again this context that will determine whether the narrator purports to convey the story as a diagnosis, a legal verdict, the fall of self or a cry for sympathy. Narratives thus are told at many levels—the personal, dialogical and social. All these levels provide an interpretive framework through which life is made meaningful and legible.

Role of the Researcher

Oftentimes for a naïve narrative researcher coming from positivistic tradition it is difficult to fathom how much his or her own individuality, background and orientation influence the construction of the illness narratives. Such influences are often involuntary, despite their effort to be neutral during the storytelling by the sick person. The researcher's stance is important in creating an environment in which a narrative is initially received and themes of inquiry conceived. The very presence of the researcher, the kind of queries and comments being made, nonverbal expressions and implicit feedback may have influence on storytelling. Narrative research thus places greater responsibility on the researcher to make explicit the lens they use in understanding and interpreting the narratives.

The initial contacts between the researcher and the narrator are crucial in forming a bond of trust and sharing. In narrative research, the interview session begins with an open-ended question, such as 'tell me something about yourself?' or 'when or how did you fall sick?' Stuhlmiller (2001) states that how the researcher responds both verbally and nonverbally to the first answer provides the narrator with a sense of the emotional climate of the interview. This appraisal in important for the narrator to decide about the nature and direction of self-disclosure he or she is willing to make. The interpersonal transaction between the researcher and the narrator is directly related to the quality and quantity of information revealed.

Understandably, listening to one's experience of being ill, a researcher needs to be empathic. A narrative researcher should be a good listener and should know how to facilitate opening up of the narrator. An empathic understanding of illness is illustrated in the work of Broyard (1992), who published accounts of illness of his narrators. He used narration to show how patients make sense of the disruption caused by illness in their lives. Broyard who himself died of cancer wrote, ... story telling seems to be a natural reaction to illness. People bleed stories, and I've become a blood bank of them (p. 20).

Another important attribute of the researcher is called 'reflexivity' in the current lexicon of qualitative research. Reflexivity requires a researcher to be constantly in reflective and self-critical mode at all stages of the research (Grbich, 2004). In other words, it involves viewing own-self vis-à-vis the process of data collection and its interpretation in a critical and informed manner. It requires a continuous inner dialogue and constant (and intensive) scrutiny of 'what I know' and 'how I know it' (Hertz, 1997, p. viii) on the part of the researcher.

Analysis of Illness Narratives

As suggested by Smith (2004) analysis of the narrative stories can be divided into two broad phases. These are descriptive and interpretive phases. In both the phases, a thorough reading and rereading of the narrative accounts is very important. It is important to identify the key features, subthemes, context and intention of the narrator. In the descriptive phase, the language usage, major themes and narrative linkages that connect different parts, the characters and roles are some aspects of the narrative scripts to which the attention is given. The second interpretive phase is rather more crucial and complex. The purpose is to identify what the narrator is trying to communicate and what sense the story makes to the narrator and the researcher and where these two perspectives converge. The whole idea is to stay with the narrative while making sense from the narrator's perspective. This task requires sensitivity and self-reflectivity on the part of researcher to derive intelligible understanding. Sometimes the researcher can also involve the participants in the process of narrative analysis.

The analysis within these two phases will depend on what question the researcher intends to take up in narrative research. Is it the structure, form or the content? Is it what the story is about or why is the story told in a particular way? Early work on the analysis of narratives is associated with the Russian Formalist School who studied folk tales and children's stories to establish a pattern of construction of a story. They divided the narrative into two essential elements—the story and the plot. The story was the sequence of action and events as they actually happened and plots were stories that were told. The formalist thus focused on uncovering universal metastructures, which underlie all narratives.

Similarly, Labov and Waletzky (1997) analysed the structure of narratives using an approach that followed these steps. First, the abstract or summary of the story was drawn, then orientation of the story (that is the time, place, situation and participants were described), complicating actions in sequence were tweezed out followed by a resolution of the story depicting what finally happened in the story. The last step involved a coda or return to the present, considering past events and depiction of an outlook for the future.

Other than the structural analysis, there is also an analysis of the content of narratives. Ricoeur (1991), as a phenomenologist, concentrated on the content of experiences rather than its structure. His analysis is thus far less a reductionist analysis strategy than that of the proponents of structural analysis.

A synthesized approach is to study the narratives in terms of both structure and content. An example of which is Stevens and Doerr's (1997) study on women's response to being infected with HIV. Their way of analysis can be summarized as beginning with an identification of a story to be analysed in the narratives, analysing the context and content of the stories with a particular focus on feelings and personal meanings, examining the consequences of diagnosis for each, and then comparing and contrasting the stories for similarities and differences. The last step involved in recognizing the effect of age, socioeconomic background on construal of experience and checking whether these add on to the previous analysis. In such an instance, both the form and content of narratives are analysed. For example, in some of our earlier works, where the main goal was to establish linkages between recovery from chronic illness and socio-cultural beliefs, we had the following broad categories for content analysis.

1. *Central theme:* What is the major concern emerging from the stories? What is the major focus in the story: people, events or disease? Whether the main theme is positive self-presentation, absolving own-self from any blame, or restoring sense of efficacy and control in the face of a long-term disease?

2. *Positive or negative orientation:* The narrative approach provided considerable flexibility to the patient to construe the health situation negatively or positively. The contents of the stories can be screened to identify preponderance of negative or positive statements. This would show whether a person has positive or negative orientation his/her illness, and life in general.

3. *Emotion-focused or problem-focused:* The narrative should reveal the nature of the perceived threat due to an illness. It is considered enduring or transient? What is the coping mechanism employed? Is the focus on management of emotions, particularly anxieties, or

focus is on dealing with the options of getting well and participating in the treatment process?

4. *Causal search:* The question which is relevant here is that does the person spontaneously engage in search for the causes of his/her illness. A ready acceptance of the suffering or invoking cultural explanations (such as Karma) would lead to ready acceptance of the suffering, rather than causal search. The nature of the recovery attributions would throw light on action orientation of the person.

5. *Behavioural stability:* Do the person consistently respond to their illness in similar manner, or that their coping pattern changes at different stages of the illness? How are the changes in emotional state linked with their behavioural stability?

6. *Repeated patterns:* This refers to recurring events or sequence of events and experiences in a specific pattern over time. It refers to repeated experiences, expressions, events or activities that reflect identifiable pattern within or across contexts, as well, across groups.

Thematic analysis: Thematic analysis is a poorly demarcated, rarely acknowledged, yet a widely used qualitative analytic method within psychology (Braun and Clarke, 2006). Thematic analysis can be employed to make sense of structure, content and process of narrative stories at the same time. Thematic analysis provides a flexible, rich and detailed, yet complex account of life stories.

Analysis involves a constant moving back and forward between the entire data set, the coded extracts of data that is being analysed, identifying the recurring themes, and then integrating them into major themes to examine and understand what narrated stories convey. A theme is understood as a recurring pattern of response or meaning with the analysed narrative(s).

More precisely, thematic analysis has the following phases:

1. Familiarizing with the narrative data by reading and rereading the scripts.

2. Generating initial codes: Coding interesting features of the scripts in a systematic manner across the entire data set, collating data relevant to each code.

3. Searching for themes: Collating codes into potential themes, gathering all data relevant to each potential theme.

4. Reviewing themes: Checking if the themes are appropriate in relation to the coded extracts (level 1) and the entire data set (level 2), generating a thematic 'map' of the analysis.

5. Defining and naming themes: Ongoing analysis to refine the specifics of each theme, and the overall story the analysis tells, generating clear definitions and names for each theme.

The themes derived through thematic analysis are sometimes arranged at four levels, namely, descriptive themes, central themes (second-order, third-order) and core themes. The themes can be arranged to form a hierarchy with descriptive themes at the base, a core theme at the apex, and two levels of central themes (second-order, third-order) in between. In this, descriptive themes are formed from the summarized meaning units of the transcribed narratives in the participant's everyday language. Second-order (central) themes are formed by reducing two or more descriptive themes. Third-order (central) themes are formed by merging two or more themes into a single one. Efforts in deriving second- and third-order (central) themes are to reduce redundancy as much as possible. Core themes are formed by reducing all of the third-order themes, with shared commonalties, to a single theme. A core theme is the central phenomenon around which all the other themes are integrated (Rennie et al., 1988). Core themes are determined by their conceptual relationship to the subsidiary themes and by their level of abstraction.

Thematic analysis is a flexible approach to analyse narrative stories across a wide range of areas and research questions. Its full potential is yet to be harnessed for in-depth analysis and generating unanticipated insights about people and their world.

Ethical Considerations in Narrative Research

In most of the traditional methods of research, even though the responses from the respondents are taken individually, in the final analysis their responses only contribute to the aggregate data. The statistical generalizations further do away with the uniqueness of the individual responses and thus ensure complete anonymity to the respondents in the research reports.

Obviously, such anonymity is not possible in narrative research, where the stories people tell are often quoted verbatim. These are the real life stories of the real people. Through their life stories, the very personal experiences of the respondents become part of the scientific writings. As these stories are used to illustrate the kind of illness experiences people have, these are presented with all details to demonstrate the relationship between specific stories and socio-cultural beliefs (for example). Frequently research participants recognize themselves in the scientific report. The readers who know these participants personally would also recognize them. This could happen even when as a routine practice names and places are disguised. This is a major ethical challenge in narrative research.

Some of such ethical challenges posed by the unique nature of narrative research are discussed here.

1. *Free and informed consent:* The principle of informed consent implies that the prior consent to interview is sought by providing all relevant information (including the aim and process of the research) and the manner in which participant's narratives are made use of. These principles, however, become problematic in narrative inquiry as it is often difficult to anticipate what will happen during the interview. By virtue of its emergent or exploratory/discovery-based approach, significant methodological decisions often are made on the spot (Price, 1996), depending upon the circumstances with each individual participant.

   What then is the alternative to such an ethical dilemma? One way out perhaps is replacing the static, standardized, one-time consent to securing, with what is called as process consent. Process consent is the act of gaining consent as a mutually negotiated process that is ongoing throughout the course of the research as compared with a consent obtained just at the outset (Balfour, 1999). Such process consent gives participants throughout the narrative process the right to reveal as much as they like and the ability to withdraw any moment they feel.

2. *Privacy and anonymity:* Both the privacy and anonymity remain problematic in the case of narrative research, which is laden with extremely private and individualistic information. This issue is resonated in McLeod's (1996) terms, where he remarked that

narratives are so 'saturated with identifying markers' (p. 311) that disguising the identities of research participants becomes a challenge. This also becomes very apparent to the participants who 'easily recognize themselves in our texts and readers who know them may recognize them, too, even when pseudonyms and other forms of disguise are used' (Chase, 1996, p. 45).

This becomes a point of major concern when narratives deal with sensitive topics like narratives of psychological counselling and health care (Balfour, 1999). The extensive use of individual stories in narrative research renders participants more vulnerable to public exposure than in traditional methods. Their health problems and the subsequent crisis no longer remain personal. It may embarrass the respondents, make them ashamed or anxious and may affect their social relationships. There may be an apprehension that their vulnerabilities may be exploited by others in different ways.

It thus becomes incumbent on narrative researchers to take steps to protect their participants from any psychological discomfort as well as undue exploitation in the process of telling their stories. Making the participants aware of the highly revelatory power of narratives can prepare them to narrate what they want to. Also, it is the duty of the researcher to judiciously share life stories of the participants with others, and that too with the participant's consent.

3. *Narrative ownership:* One ethical issue that resonates especially in narrative research concerns the ownership of narratives. That is, who has the final control and authority over presentation and interpretation of the narratives? In narratives, it assumes an important dimension and the question arises that can one simply give away one's story, especially when it is so heavily invested with one's personal meaning and sense of identity?

This issue becomes even more pertinent when participants of a narrative study react to researchers' analyses of their stories with scepticism and a sense of betrayal. It is commonly reported that the final analysis done by the researcher fails to capture experiences fully in all its uniqueness and individuality. Such reactions are perhaps inevitable in instances where people's stories are transformed into instances of larger social or psychological phenomena.

There is a possibility that the researcher might approach a life story from a different perspective than the individual who tells the story. Chase (1996) addressed the matter in the following way:

Who should control the interpretive process in any particular case depends in large part on the aim or purpose of the research and thus what kind of material needs to be collected and what kind of interpretation best suits that material. Moreover, as long as decisions about these questions are made by the researcher ... the researcher continues to exercise authority not shared with participants.... I believe that claiming and acknowledging one's interpretive authority is imperative. (pp. 51–52)

The above discussion points out that there seems to be no simple solution to these ethical dilemmas, which a researcher faces in narrative research.

10

Self-construal among Healthy and Chronically Sick Women*

For centuries, women in India identified themselves with their roles as daughters, wives and mothers. They have conformed to role-specific responsibilities and expectations, and by the ideals prescribed for them by the society. They remained rooted in social-affiliative system, confining and conforming to a network of social relationships, and thus maintaining the stability of society's cultural institutions (Parikh & Garg, 1989). The aspirations and activities of these Indian women remained family-centred, as they sacrifice their personal needs to fulfill larger social obligations. Though all along the history, women were part of the work force, engaged in a wide range of activities in the outside world, the society continued to identify them with their familial roles only. Literature, religion and cultural lore eulogized women who lived by the virtues of their social role expectations. Women defined and crystallized their self-identity only in relation to their families. Against this backdrop this study examined the role of health status in organizing women's self-construal. The main objective of the study was to understand how chronically sick women who hail from

* Published in Dalal, A.K. and Biswas, G. (2009). Self-construal among healthy and chronically sick women. *Psychological Studies, 54*(2), 142–149.

Mrs Gita Biswas is a consultant and programme evaluator for NGO in the area of Women and Family. This text has been edited for typographical errors, stylistic consistency, and sequential organization in order to make it suitable for inclusion in this book.

the urban-middle-class families background construe their self-identity, discover themselves in different social roles, while dealing with the vicissitudes of every-day life. A comparative analysis of the constructions of self of healthy and sick women was undertaken to provide insights into their struggle to retain a positive self-image in a rapidly changing traditional society.

The contours of the world in which Indian women have lived so far are rapidly changing in recent times. Socioeconomic changes, as well as, global exposures through television and telecommunication are now heralding new possibilities and new images of womanhood for them. Educated, armed with skills and knowledge, today's woman is rediscovering herself beyond the confines of existing social structures and networks of relationship. 'Like their male counterparts, they enter into the world of occupation, career, profession, competition and achievements in their own right and create a space where the need to experience themselves and be accepted as autonomous beings is dominated' (Parikh & Garg, 1989, p. 25). Even those who are circumscribed by their social roles are also feeling a pressure from within and without to give a new meaning to their self-identity. They never had so much space and freedom to vision themselves in newer roles, beyond the boundaries which society had imposed on them (Chatterji, 1997).

Today, Indian women are caught in cross-currents of a culture in transition. She is facing a major challenge of balancing a traditional and a modern world in her life. The gains of modernization in terms of social liberalism and individual emancipation are at times offset by the negative aspects of the devaluation of the human qualities in urban India (Menon, 2004). Also, the pursuit of independence and achievements creates guilt at not fulfilling the traditional role, anxieties about their inadequacy and apprehensions of being accused or ridiculed. Their lives have already become a battleground between the prescriptive roles based on idealized past and a dream of the future of autonomy and independence. This conflict in internalized more often by educated, urban middle class women. Ghadially (1988), Seymour (1999) and Davar (1998) have discussed at length this dilemma which Indian women are facing today.

Unable to resolve the duality of their existence, many of these women are caught in mid-life crises. Their husbands want them to be traditional at home and modern in public; their children seek nurturance but resent indulgence; they work in office and carry domestic chorus without much support. She is grown up, mature and worldly wise, but is at the same time conscious of the widening gap between her dream image of herself and the real one (Channa, 1997). This is the stage in life when a woman is prone to engaged in self-appraisal and self-reflective exercises.

A woman reaching mid-life has to confront the reality that youth and womanhood has started receding into the past. She is no longer centre of gravity for her husband and children who get busy in their own worlds. As Parikh and Garg (1989) observed, though she is now in a very familiar and predictable surrounding, there is a strange sense of being lost. Many women find it hard to let go their long-cherished dreams of a purposeful life and suffer from a feeling of meaningless existence. They become indecisive and confused, angry and reactive, and frustrated, realizing that there is no escape from the expectations of the familial world they were caught in. In a study (Singh & Singh, 1999) many of the middle-aged school teachers reported that they were not able to perform now their work with same efficiency as earlier. It causes anxiety and irritation, many times results in unpleasantness with husband and children. It was found that more than three-fourth of the sample expressed negative feelings of depression, frustration, loneliness, anxiety and fear about their aging. Chatterji (1997) reported that health of these women remain neglected because she has never learnt to pay attention to her own well-being.

Many of her conflicts which she had buried in the turbulent period of establishing herself as a wife, mother and daughter-in-law resurfaces, as she can no longer hold her 'self' in abeyance. She sees a danger of her real self-being engulfed by the social networks. In such instances one possibility is that her aggression towards husband and in-laws turn inward, against her own self and internalize cultural devaluation of women as her own feelings of worthlessness and inferiority. Basu (1995) found greater deal of discrepancy in self in the case of middle-age Bengali women. Isaac and Shah (2004) found that Indian women are less satisfied with their own self and accomplishments. Though, they may find some compensatory reward in their motherhood and in the achievements of their children.

As Peterson et al. (1988) found in their work that mid-life (35 to 45 years of age) is the most vulnerable age to catch health problems. They conducted a 35-year-long follow-up study to establish linkages between negative mental states and physical health. As they discovered, in the young age when physical health is robust, it is not much affected by her mental state. As they enter mid-life, their attitudes and expectations play crucial role in shaping their physical health status. People who are pessimistic and helpless are more likely to get into variegated health problems. Those who could find space to express their individuality, or make sense of their social position could be those who remain healthy. In other words, there seems to be a close symbiotic relationship between self-construal and physical health status.

It is posited in this study that women's self-construal is a dynamic entity, not just an end product in terms of a given structure. Self-construal is the inclusion of elements of social world in one's self definition (Markus & Kitayama, 1991). The self in this sense is not what one is, but is a system of internalizing social values and traditions. It arises in social interactional process and the manner in which social experiences and events are being interpreted by a person. Gergen and Gergen (1988) have argued that such social construal of self serves as a referent to make sense of ongoing life experiences and events. This is a process through which people come to understand their own selves and the social world they live in. Such self-construal denotes what they think they are and determine their relationships and participation in social life. This bidirectional causality keeps the self socially grounded, as a relatively stable and continuous entity. More importantly in the present context, it affects and gets affected by one's health status.

Chronic health experience often tempers with woman's self-image. For some it could be a respite from facing hard realities of the life; for others it erodes their sense of respect and self-worth. Her body image and social relationship are undermined by the fact that she is no longer provider of nurturance and care to their family members. It would be enlightening to examine how their material, social and spiritual selves act and interact with each other to compensate for the chronic sickness. The illness, indeed, provides an opportunity to probe deeper into the inner world of a woman.

While attempting to understand women's construal of their own-self, it is important to use appropriate method which had potential to probe into her personal world. An appropriate method is that which can go into the depths of her psyche and can provide an understanding of her existential dilemmas. Parikh and Garg (1989) discovered in their dialogue with more than 2000 women that a women rarely talks about herself. She mostly talks about her social roles, her family and social networks. She may talk about her personal observations once for a while, but keeps her intimate feelings to herself.

Under these conditions, narrative method was found to be the most appropriate choice. Narratives of the lived life experiences are the means to communicating and detailing their lives to others. The way people construct and communicate their life stories is often conditioned by culturally available resources and by the images of their own-self (Williams, 2000). Life narratives thus can be very rich source of material to enhance our understanding of the self and social world of Indian women, as they are impacted by their health status. These narratives are examined and understood without any preconceived categories and theoretical frameworks.

In the narrative approach as employed in this study, without taking recourse to any prepared questionnaire, women were encouraged to free associate with their important life events and share them with the researcher. In informal sessions, these women were asked about their personal experiences, feelings and actions. They were encouraged to reflect back in identifying salient influences on their lives. A narrative construction of personal experiences and events was what constituted research data.

In the present study narratives of healthy and chronically sick women were collected and interpreted to establish the potent role of health status in defining and designing one's self-identity.

Method

Participants

The study was conducted on 10 healthy and 10 chronically sick women. Healthy women were those who did not have any health problem (except seasonal ailments, like cough, cold) in the past 5 years. The chronically sick were those who suffered one or the other health problem in the same period. Most of the sick women in this study had problems, like peptic ulcer, colitis, spondalitis and high blood pressure. They were constantly under treatment for their illness, causing frequent disruption in their daily routine.

Table 10.1:
Demographic background of healthy and chronically sick women

Demographic Background	Healthy	Sick
Mean age (in years)	36.7	37.6
Years of marriage (in years)	15.6	17.9
Education		
Senior school	1	3
Graduation	7	4
Master's degree	2	3
Work status		
Employed	5	3
Housewife	5	7
No. of children (mean)	2.1	2.2

These women participants belonged to urban, middle-class families from Allahabad, India. Their age ranged between 35 and 40 years. They were married for at least 10 years and were living with their husbands, children and in-laws. All of them were educated—a majority of them studied up to graduation and post-graduation. Eight of these women were employed, rest were house-wives. All of them hailed from traditional, upper caste family background, belonging to middle income group. Most of them were from the Bengali community. The demographic breakup of the participants is given in Table 10.1. Care was taken to select the women who were willing to reflect and share their life experiences.

Narrative Sessions

Narrative sessions were conducted in the home setting. The second author of this paper visited these women with prior appointment. The preferred meeting time used to be before forenoon when other members of the family were busy elsewhere. The idea was to have some privacy and enough time to engage in conversation. These meetings were not for the purpose of any formal interview, but for what we called 'informal chat sessions'. Some demographic information was obtained at the initial stage, as well as, information about the nature of illness was sought from the chronically sick women. The purpose of the interview was made clear as to know about their life experiences, particularly, to talk about their health experiences. There was no fixed agenda or interview schedule to elicit responses. The researchers only had a list of questions to guide the inquiry. An environment of trust, understanding and friendship was cultivated during the initial contacts. Since the researcher also belonged to the same age, social class and family background, it was easier to establish a trusting relationship. She talked about her own life experiences, family and health problems to be an active participant in the conversation. This mostly worked well in soliciting cooperation of the respondents.

In subsequent sessions, the respondents were encouraged to reflect on their health experiences. What major changes have occurred in their lives in the past 5 years? What does good health mean to them? How has illness experience changed their lives? The respondents were encouraged to go into their past, think about the major events and their responses to them. Those who were sick were asked to think in terms of their illness experiences. The researcher minimally intervened to maintain the conversational flow.

In fact, the researchers as well as the respondents had no prior experience of conducting such narrative inquiry. The first three respondents were taken as practice cases and were dropped from the study. A thorough discussion with colleagues on what really transpired in these practice encounter gave confidence to researcher in handling health narratives. Again, as we discovered, all the respondents were naïve in the sense that they had no prior experience of this kind of reflective exercise. Many of these women found it difficult to talk about their personal lives and often avoided talking about themselves directly. They instead talked about other people in their lives. They opened up only in subsequent sessions. The most difficult topic to talk about was husband–wife relationship. There was, of course, variation in self-disclosure of these women. The researcher took detailed noted of whatever respondents said and filled the gaps in subsequent sessions.

It took three to five sessions with each respondent to get all the information for this study. The respondents were helped to re-examine and re-evaluate the incidences of their lives. For some it was an emotional reliving of the traumatic experiences and cried while narrating their experiences. In such cases, the researcher had to double up as a counselor. On an average, the researcher spent about 8–10 hours with each respondent.

Results and Discussion

Each narrative was read and re-read by both coauthors of this paper to make sense of health narratives of the participants. The main focus was on understanding, how the construal of self differed for healthy and chronically sick women. We looked for the emerging themes and patterns of narrations across all healthy women and compared these patterns with those of the sick women. We focused only on those patterns of narrative scripts which were coherent and consistent, indicative of some salient features of self perception. We could identify some recurring themes that formed the basis of interpreting these narratives.

Location of Identity

Location here means the position from which a woman views herself. It is the reference point from which she comprehends her appearance, relationships, virtues, deficiencies and her life as a woman. Though some of these women described themselves in terms of professional, physical and social attributes, their predominant identity was that of a mother. It is in the motherhood that they find meaning and purpose of their living. A typical self-description follows as:

> I am a teacher and a mother of two daughters. I live with my husband, children and in-laws. I have a small house that I try to keep clean and tidy.

Another self-description of a healthy housewife shows similar pattern:

> I am his wife. I have many positive attributed in me. I am mother of two daughters. When I watch TV and realize that women can do a lot, I feel that if I had learnt good tailoring I would have started my own business.

There are though few differences in the narratives of healthy and sick women. One, in the case of sick women there is greater assertion of individuality. They see themselves as a person and maintain a self-object distinction. They are conscious of their appearance. For example, here is self-description of a women suffering from chronic gastric condition:

> *I am ... I am graduate, a teacher. I am happy go-lucky. I am a tall, fair complexioned, black haired woman. Singing is my hobby. I like clean surrounding, tidy home. I do cleaning, washing, all myself.* (Asha)

She is the women who had gone through a very turbulent period. Both she and her husband were short tempered and never got along well. Her husband had high blood pressure and during one of their verbal fight, he got very excited and had the attack of paralysis. He was admitted in the hospital and doctors lost hopes of his recovery. 'I was completely stunned but did not cry. I kept praying to the God and nursed him without failure. He recovered in three months time. Now I do not get so much angry but often cry silently. I am very much worried about my children. If something happens to me, who will take care of them. It depresses me'.

Another sick woman who is not happy with her life conditions was not interested in talking about herself. She had suffered from multiple illnesses, was withdrawn and her elder daughter was managing most of the household work.

> *My name is ... I am a housewife. I don't do anything, so there is no point in talking about myself any further.*

Its contrast a healthy women considered herself a woman first and a wife later. She is second wife of a doctor and is herself a nurse by profession who viewed herself in a larger social context. Her positive construal is evident in what she had to say about herself.

> *I am a woman, wife of a doctor. I am a nurse by profession but a social worker by activities. I enjoy helping people in trouble and try to connect with them. I never think of future and am happy with what I am doing.*

Another self-introduction of a happy and healthy woman,

> *I belong to a middle class family. I am an ordinary person, considered myself a happy and successful housewife. I am lucky to have got a good family in marriage that care for me. I am only worried about the education of my three children.*

Gender-specific Imageries

The self-image which most of these women had of themselves centered around traditional social roles. The images imprinted in their minds were those of nearest familial roles—that of mother and wife—not of the generalized role base on gender differentiation. However, in all these women a yearning to be unconventional was clearly noticeably. The sick women were, indeed torn between these two contradictory demands. Self-doubt, uncertainty, fear, confusion and other such typical symptoms characterize the self-imagery of these women. On the other hand, physically healthy women were able to strike balance and harmony between these two opposite desires. These women were able to perceive themselves as a unit of a larger social system and their self-concept hinged on a broader domain. The two narratives given here highlight this contrast.

I got married at an early age and had three children one after another. Even then I could complete my studies with family support. My in-laws are also living with us and we all live happily. For me family well-being is foremost and always feed husband and children first. I easily make friends and win trust of others. (Manisha)

Women of poor health had different stories to tell. One of them said:

Wife is devalued in our society. She is burdened with responsibilities and has to tolerate too much in her life. If she does not adjust herself to the demands of her family after marriage she will not be at peace. Her life is suffering and worse, she is not supposed to open her mouth. She suffers silently and faces the consequences. Bengali women, like me, are expected to serve without caring for their health.

Other respondent, Vibha, suffered from peptic ulcer and was hospitalized frequently. She was a housewife and considered it a curse. She observed,

Women keep doing their domestic work till they fall sick. They ignore their disease and hide it till it is intolerable. We have to do strenuous work that is why our illness takes serious turn. I had to please everyone after marriage. In my middle age I had a feeling that I had tortured myself enough.

For the women who were chronically sick, motherhood was not a rewarding or growth experience but is seen as a compensation for her sacrifices. Their sense of achievement is reflected in the achievements of their children. If the children are not doing well, it aggravates their personal crises. For healthy women, children's performance is one of the many sources of life satisfaction.

Themes of Uprooting

One of the major turning points in lives of all these women was marriage, and more than that to leave their own families and to settle in a place and among people which were unfamiliar. It was like replanting themselves in an entirely new environment. The themes of such uprooting are very much evident in all the narratives.

For the women who were healthy, this transition was smooth and growth oriented. They succeed in building a bridge between the two worlds and could freely move from one side to the other. They were accepted by their in-laws with whom they forged a new relationship. One healthy woman mentioned,

> *We are four brothers and sisters. I got lot of love from my mother. She gave me good upbringing. After marriage, husband and in-laws took good care of me. Outside people think that I take too much attention to maintain my health. My husband thinks that I don't do much for my health.* (Vinati)

On the contrary, sense of uprooting is a major theme in the narratives of sick women. When Sharda (name changed) was asked about the saddest time in her life, she mentioned unhesitatingly that was when she realized that her in-laws place was worse than her worst dreams. She stated,

> *I am least satisfied with my present. There is a big difference in parents house and here—in status, food habits, life style. Here they use abusive language. I had too many problems in adjusting after marriage. My husband is good—he is different. We finally got separated from the in-laws.*

Meenakshi's story is a case in point. Her both parents and brother had died in the recent past. She only had distant relatives in her father's house, no one in particular to receive her. She still crave to return to her father's house. As she narrated:

> *Last year my brother died. Same month father died. Mother died later on. I was youngest in the family and I can't forget all of them. This brother gave me blood when I was sick earlier. I always crave to go to my father's house.*

In contrast, a healthy woman stated that the worst day in her life was when her sister-in-law died young and she could not do much. Many of these healthy women viewed their marriage as a practical solution to their many life crises. They accepted their present state more sanguinely. Some of these healthy women maintained their close ties with their own family and did not suffer separation. As Meera said:

> *My husband works in other city and comes home in holidays only. I mostly stay with my parents and it works well in my case. I don't miss him*

World of Relationships

Indian women live in a complex web of relationship. They define their identity in terms of relationships. They derive their energy, their vitality from these relationships. These are the close family relationships which are both—the source of pain and pleasure for middle-aged Indian house-wives.

In case of sick women, their relationship with husband and in-laws are always very difficult. There was no evidence to suggest that these women tried to patch up with their in-laws or tried to smoother the relationship, instead the endeavour was to make life a little more tolerable. There is a changing view of husband from indifferent, coercive to that of a little more tolerant person. The healthy women find it easy to form new relationships and find meaning in them.

Kavita who got married at a very young age found herself much settled in her relationships with her in-laws and husband. In her words:

> *People say I keep very good health despite age and grown up children. Still my old fashioned mother-in-law feels concerned about my health and keeps saying that I am week and need to gain some weight. I was strongly attached to me sister-in-law who died few years back. I always regret that I could not do much for her. My*

mother-in-law and daughters take full responsibility of running the household. I get enough time to read books and play harmonium.

It was quite different experience for Nisha who was teaching in a school and suffered many health problems.

My health problem began with the illness of my son and got aggravated after his death. I stopped taking care of my health, stopped eating properly. In my in-laws house I had to serve every one, a difficult task. I had problem with my husband whose carelessness forced me to abort thrice. My unemployed brother is another source of concern for me.

What comes out from the narratives is that whereas, sick women have a feeling of being stuck up in a relationship, healthy women experience a sense of autonomy. They succeed in carving out a social space for themselves where they can experiment and innovate, and feel their individuality. Vinati likes to visit her friends, Kavita is active in a local NGO, Manisha participates in drama and music competition. The story of Kamla who had a serious health problem in the previous year is rather different.

I was down with rheumatic fever and was hospitalized. My mother-in-law and daughter attended me but my husband did not come to see me. He was annoyed that now he has to spend a good amount of money on my treatment. My husband is attached to his mother and I know nothing about his job, I feel in shackles here.

A significant indicator of health and sickness was the relationship with in-laws. Wherever, these relations were strained, health became a major casualty. The themes of being harassed and exploited by in-laws were frequent. Most of these women saw their husband as different from the rest of the family. Kunti who broke away from her husband's joint family after years of recriminations separated and suffered chronic headache stated:

I am not satisfied. It is just sort of o.k., Their (in-laws') behaviour was not what I had expected. There was a big difference in social status, eating habits and living style. Because of all this I faced a lot of problems. And then, after 7 years I got separated from my in-laws. But my husband is a very nice human being. His temperament does not match with anyone in his family. His thinking and friend circle are very different.

This is a healthy woman:

After marriage I got the cooperation and affection of every one, particularly of father and mother-in-laws. I have more freedom here than I had at my mother's place. I never indulge in a situation which may lead to tension. When I get angry, my husband lightens up the whole situation.

Tradition vs. Modernity

Respondents taken in the study seemed to have caught in social transition, trying to balance between the two worlds of tradition and modernity. The demands of these two worlds are different, each pulling the respondents in opposing direction. Whereas modernity calls for independent, self-contained and autonomous mode of self, traditional self is emotionally bound to family and relations. For her personal needs and desires are subordinate to collective interest of the family. Traditional values call for sacrificing personal well-being before family. Thus whereas traditional model lays emphasizes on social roles (e.g. motherhood) and interdependence, modernity promoted ego-centric functioning of self, the emphasis is on personal achievements and carrier, and builds around individuated selfhood. Thus, whereas traditional self is other-focused, modernity is self-focused. Indian women struggle to reconcile these opposing forces of traditional ideals and modern aspirations in her psyche (Kakar & Kakar, 2007). These two opposing pulls within these women create stress and conflicts, and have implications for their health status. The narratives revealed that healthy and sick women differed in their resolution to this dilemma. In general, it was observed that whereas healthy women made no efforts to resolve this dichotomy and accepted it as part of living, for the sick this transition proved oppressive and they strived to resolve it.

For most of the healthy respondents life was an orderly transition from one stage to another. They were more tied with the traditional roles and tried to contain their ambitions and greater concern about mental freedom. Many of them believed in the theory of karma and took the life as it came. Though they were craving for freedom and wanted to assert their individuality, they were able to dwell in both the worlds. The sick respondents thought the other way round.

Those who could not fulfill their needs and wishes, like me, tend to fall sick. I was very adventurous before marriage, now nobody appreciates what I do. My son had a hole in the heart. Relations and neighbours kept advising me what to do. It delayed the treatment and my son died. (Vibha)

Believe in God and accept His judgment. I keep worshiping all the time. But my mind wanders and keep asking 'why me? Why do I have to suffer so much? (Meenakshi)

Sharing and Self-disclosure

Most of the healthy people shared their happiness but not sorrow. They did not share when no solution was in sight. They often shared with their daughters, husband or some friend, as two excerpts given below show.

I share my health problems with everyone—husband, children and in-laws. I can't tolerate when someone ignores me. When my husband, children do not attend to my illness I get very irritated.

The other group of narratives is characterized by low sharing and low self-disclosure. These are from the narratives of four respondents who preferred to keep their suffering to themselves.

I sit alone and brood. Never share my problems with anyone. They are very personal. What's point in sharing it when no one can do anything about it.

I have grudges but no one to talk to. Keep them to myself.

I share only with my daughters. Husband has no time for me; he is not interested in listening anything. In fact, when I talk to him about some problem, he loses his patience and starts shouting.

Share happiness with husband and daughters. I do not share my unhappiness with anyone, except to God and cry before Him. I share with my neighbour. She is my guardian and friend. I feel light after talking to her.

This finding that the sick women are lower on sharing and self-disclosure than the healthy women is understandable. Siegel (1991) had noted, 'When you put your feelings outside, you may heal inside. And you will certainly heal your life, if not your disease; for emotional repression prevents the healing system from responding as a unified entity to threats from inside or outside' (p. 188). Pennebaker (1991) also opined that sharing one's true feelings and needs helps one to unlock the power of one's healing system. Anger, anxiety, depression, fear and many other feelings are unhealthy when they remain buried inside, unexpressed and not dealt with.

Concluding Comments

This narrative study of married, middle-aged Indian women has clearly evinced that chronically sick and healthy women differ in their self-construal. Healthy people were accepting of their life conditions and had a relatively stable notion about their own-self. They were more in tune with their familial environment and more often resorted to positive construction of themselves and of the negative life events. Healthy women found it easier to relate with people within their social world and at the same time could carve out a personal domain in which they were free to experiment. They could garner a high self-esteem as their self was better grounded in social relationships. On the contrary, there was greater turbulence in the lives of sick women and they were not able to reconcile with the discrepancy in their ideal and actual self; between dreams and reality. Their lives were much more eventful and they had lot to narrate. They are fighting more with themselves than with the external world. These were the women who were fighting against their destiny and are not prepared to accept their fate. Poor health is the cost which they had paid for asserting their individuality and trying to control own lives and that of others. The sick women rebelled but suffered their agony without much sharing. This comparative scenario profile of healthy and sick women is, of course, not uniform and show general trend.

11

Family Support and Coping with Chronic Diseases*

Falling sick is a family event in India. It not only affects well-being of the patient but also of the whole family; disrupting the normal routine and adjustment of other family members. Depending on the nature and severity of the sickness, the family is required to mobilize its internal and external resources to cope with the impending crisis. Additional demands and responsibilities are shared by the family members to provide physical and emotional support to facilitate patient's recovery and return to normal routine. Family treatment and care are important predictors of successful coping with many diseases. On the basis of his work in India and China, Kleinman (1974) observed that more than 80% of all sickness are managed within family and its extended network, without resorting to professional help from outside.

The role of family is more salient in the case of chronic diseases, such as rheumatic heart, arthritis, asthma and diabetes for various reasons. First, a strong relationship exists between family and illness; chronic illness affects and is affected by the family context. Family interaction and living pattern engenders many life stresses resulting in high susceptibility to a number of diseases. Some families, thus, have a high frequency of falling sick. At the same time, the characteristic manner in which the

* Published in Dalal, A.K. (1995). Family support and coping with chronic diseases. *Indian Journal of Social Work, 46,* 167–176.
  This text has been edited for typographical errors, stylistic consistency, and sequential organization in order to make it suitable for inclusion in this book.

family appraises illness of its member, decides about the treatment regimen and provides emotional support influences the sickness outcomes. Second, a chronic disease needs long-term and sustained treatment, which is mostly home based. Thus, the way the family handles chronic sickness can very much influence the course of the disease. Third, since family support is a long-term need in case of a chronic illness (e.g. heart disease), it may require patient and other members of the family to make some enduring changes in their life routine. Many times interpersonal boundaries are redrawn in the face of a chronic problem. Fourth, more often than not, people suffering from chronic disease need emotional support to manage their own lives. They have adjustment problems and put much strain on family relationships. Whereas a short-term acute or life-threatening sickness generally brings the whole family together to put up a common front, a long-term sickness which lays relentless demands on family resources tends to tear many families apart.

It is evident from the research literature that despite all limitations and restrictions imposed by the chronic illness, most of the families do rather well to cope with the crisis. Family relationships are essentially the most important source of support that a chronically ill person can have and the positive outcomes of family support are well founded. There is, however, not much work to enlighten how the support system operates in the Indian context. When does family support help, when does it fail? Research in this domain is traditionally restricted to linear approach in which the response flow is from the family to the patient who needs treatment and support. The alternative system approach emphasizes continuous interchange among all the family members, as well as with the external environment. A family as an organic entity endures stresses of the illness of a family member; provides support though at times needs support. This article attempts to reconcile some of the contradictory research findings regarding the efficacy of the family support in coping with chronic diseases. Some criteria to identify vulnerable families will be discussed along with the implications for intervention strategies.

Family as a Primary Care Giver

In all traditional curative systems in India, family is considered to be a basic unit for health care and medical intervention. In fact, this role of primary care giver is integral to the value system of the Indian society.

As Gore (1968) and Sinha (1982) noted, India has a long history of stable family life and structure which has well survived the test of the times. Even during the most trying times of social upheavals in the past, family structure and sense of a collective responsibility have remained sustaining influence. As an institution, Indian family has shown remarkable adaptability in meeting new demands of the changing world. The research from this perspective has yielded findings which have almost idealized the Indian traditional family system in its role as a primary caregiver.

During last 3–4 decades, the country has gone through rapid socio-economic changes with large scale migration of population from rural to urban areas. Notwithstanding, it has brought only limited changes in the Indian family which still retains many of its traditional features (Sinha, 1988). It is argued that though joint family system is weakening in big cities, it is not acquiring the typical character of a nuclear family. Gupta (1978) observed that a new nuclear type family does not really exist as a separate entity, but as a sector of the continuous extended family arrangement. As Gore (1968) put it, structurally the extended family is tending to become nuclear, but functionally it is maintaining jointness. There are various economic, social and practical considerations also which predisposes the younger generation not to break away from the extended family. The transition of a joint family seems to be towards a close network of primary-kin-type nuclear families to retain the support base.

The concern about the breaking of joint families appears natural, given the overwhelming research finding that joint families provide larger support base which buffers the stresses of disease or disability (e.g. Kakar, 1982; Sethi & Sharma, 1982). Despite some contradictory evidence, the general finding that nuclear-type families have more health problems holds (Bharat, 1991). In recent years, two developments have greatly revived the interest in understanding how family support helps its members in managing chronic illness. One is increase in longevity from 32 to 59 years in last 45 years. This has resulted in greater number of cases of chronic disease. It is found that chronic disease or its complication is responsible for 75% of all the deaths worldwide (Taylor, 2006). A much larger chunk of the population now needs family care than ever before. Second factor which has put greater responsibility of care on family is the rapid decline of hospital services in India. Indian hospitals are overcrowded, lack basic amenities and are insensitive to patients' suffering. Inflated cost of treatment in health-care institutions has rendered them out of reach to a larger section of the society (Banerjee, 1993). The result is that most of the medical care of the chronic patients is outside the medical institutions; primarily within the family set-up. Family support is thus crucial in dealing with the instances of chronic sicknesses.

Family Support and Successful Coping

Family support is defined as a feeling that a person is cared about and valued by other family members and that he or she can fall back on family network in difficult times. In behavioural sense, family support refers to emotional, instrumental and financial assistance obtained from one's own family. House and Kahn (1985) distinguished among emotional support, appraisal support (affirmation, feedback, etc.), informational support and instrumental support (money, effort, etc.). The factors which relate to these types of family support are family size, living arrangement, frequency of contact, closeness of relationship, sharing responsibilities, communication pattern, etc. In this article the focus is mainly on psychosocial aspects of family support.

Research in this area in early 70s began with the broader concept of social support. A large body of research related to social support included actual and implied presence of family members and subjective appraisal of their support efforts. It is in this sense that family was taken as a primary source of social support. In fact, as House, Robbins and Metzner (1982) have argued, relationship with family members and particularly with spouse largely account for the association between social support and adaptional outcomes. Moreover, there is evidence that support from other sources does not entirely compensate for what is lacking in close relationships (Coyne & DeLongis, 1986).

The research evidence is overwhelming that social support, of which family is the most important component, can directly improve health, as well as buffer the effects of stress (Caplan, 1974; Cassel, 1976). A relationship between mental health and family support is established in many Indian studies. Bharat (1991) found in 10 out of 20 studies she reviewed that the nuclear-type families were more susceptible to psychiatric disorders than the joint families. She found contradictory evidence only in three studies. Sharma and Srivastava (1991) also arrived at a similar conclusion. They both attributed these psychiatric disorders to lack of supportive network in a nuclear-type family, in comparison to a joint family. Ramachandran et al. (1982) found that respondents over the age of 50 years from the nuclear and single-member families were more depressed than those from the joint families. Blazer (1982) also reported that greater availability, frequency and positive perception of social support in the elderly were associated with decreased mortality. Elderly people with impaired social support were three times more likely to die during the 30 months of the study than those with good social support. In this study of elderly, the presence and number of living children were the most powerful predictors of survival. In a nine-year long study on a large sample of respondents living in California, Berkman and Syme (1979) showed that a number of network and support indicators (marriage, contact with family and friends, church membership and other group affiliations) were associated with reduced mortality risk.

However, apart from this global finding that the support helps, the available research has not provided much insight into the ways in which family support plays a positive role in coping with chronic diseases. Little is known about the underlying process through which family support may affect health outcomes. Most of the earlier researches in this area have relied on correlational, retrospective and case–control designs, with very few longitudinal and intervention studies. These studies rarely took a comprehensive or standard measure of family support, rather different indices of family support were used to predict some health outcomes. It is, thus, often difficult making comparisons across studies.

There were, however, some efforts to understand the mechanism through which support affects health outcomes. It has become clear from few studies that support influences health by enhancing coping effectiveness; by changing the ways people under stress appraise their situation and respond by directing efforts to master or to adapt to the demands of the chronic illness (Gore, 1985). Emotional and social support thus protects people from deleterious effects of prolonged distress by influencing an individual's initial appraisal of the stressors, coping strategy or self-worth (Caplan, 1979; Caplan, Naidu & Tripathi, 1986; Lieberman, 1982). Lieberman (1982) also found that those who have adequate support are more likely to engage in health promoting behaviour, are less prone to develop some types of health problems, and are more likely to seek medical care than those who have low support. Caplan (1979) posited that social support increases a person's feeling of security and thus lowers his or her defensive, counterproductive coping strategies. Caplan pointed out that social support might also result in improved coping by putting more information at the disposal of the recipient, thereby increasing the accuracy of self-perception and that of the environment. The enhanced access to information through support group may motivate the person to engage in adaptive behaviours. Cobb (1979) argued that the feeling of obligation to those whom one loves may enhance motivation to adhere to difficult treatment regimen.

Often family support will interact with other variables to indirectly influence the health outcomes. The support group provides an opportunity to the patient to freely ventilate their anxieties, to arrive at a shared understanding of the disease and to explore various alternative coping strategies. Some studies have focused on 'buffering effects', or the ability of support to ameliorate the impact of chronic stress on health (Taylor, 1991). This finding is supported in many epidemiological community surveys of depressive symptoms (Sethi & Sharma, 1982; Slater & Depue, 1980). Although the evidences for stress-buffering effects of support are far from uniform, it seems that the emotional support plays a more important role in protecting the patient from the deleterious effects of stress than other contextual variables (e.g. Kessler, McLeaod & Wethington, 1984). Lack of social support makes one susceptible to develop some kind of psychopathology. Furthermore, characteristics of the recipient, provider and the setting may determine whether or not support provided is effective. For example, available family support will be beneficial only if people have social skills to mobilize help from those in their support network (Hirsch, 1981).

When Support Fails

Whereas the social support literature tends to emphasize the benefits that may accrue from helpful involvement of others, a small but growing number of clinical and life crisis studies suggests that in many instances support efforts do not have the intended outcomes. Studies on families attempting to help a member who is facing a crisis document the fallibility of family relationships as a source of support. There is evidence that while trying to provide help a partner in crisis, family members often become involved in ways that are constraining and debilitating

(Speedling, 1982). There are cases of destructive over-involvement of close relatives. These aspects of the family support are not paid much attention to.

As posited by Coyne, Wortman and Lehman (1988) there is usually a 'honeymoon' period in the case of any chronic disease which as a sudden start, like myocardial infarction or detection of malignancy. The other family members may break their normal routine, suspend other activities, become visibly more caring and forge a stronger family bond. During this period positive orientation and optimism are voiced, along with the expression of empathy and commitment to reassure the patient of family solidarity to collectively fight out the crisis. There is gradual depletion of this spirit as the crisis lingers and there are other urgent things to attend.

In many instances while trying to provide help, close family members are at times equally or even more distressed and anxious than the patient. Studies reveal that spouses of the recent heart patients are actually more distressed than the heart patients (Gillis, 1984). Thus, rather than being of help, they may cause additional anxiety in the patient. Varma (1989) found that spouses of the cancer patients go through the same stages as does the patients. These spouses, in fact, need social support to cope with their personal crisis rather than being able to provide support. St. Louis et al. (1982) found that physicians tend to believe that family members are less effective in providing cardiopulmonary resuscitation than are the persons who are emotionally detached.

The family therapy research has made enough contribution to understand how people trying to help others in distress become emotionally over-involved, critical and hostile to the stressed person. At the initial stage of a chronic disease, people rally round the patient putting aside all old conflicts, rivalries and ill-feelings. If the situation continues unabated, as in the case of chronic diseases, the help providers may feel frustrated, and in trying to take control of the events become over involved and demanding. If the help-recipient does not heed to the advice, or do things other way, the help provider may consider it as rejection of their efforts and resent. Particularly when the family health providers have made substantial investment in the recovery of the patients, they get upset if the recovery is not fast enough, or if the patient report additional complaints. In such conditions generally the attribution is that the person who is suffering is not making sufficient efforts herself or himself. Such 'blaming of the victim' is very common, making the patient more defensive. The result is that in many instances people prefer to suffer with stoic calmness, putting up a facade of all-well, till their condition seriously aggravate.

Wortman and Lehman (1985) have on the basis of the review of the existing research stated three basic reasons why people respond to the victim of life crises in the ways that are unsupportive. One, social psychological research shows that people often feel uncomfortable in the presence of those who are suffering, unhappy or in need of help. Contact with victims of chronic diseases may generate negative feelings because this shatters one's illusions of invulnerability, or because it evokes strong feeling of helplessness. In the case of close friend or family member, interactions may also elicit fears and anxieties about what lies ahead, or whether the support provider will be able to handle the increased demands that may be placed on him or her. Since such interactions could be distressing, people distance from the patient if possible, or at least discourage him or her to ventilate anxieties and worries. Consequently, individuals in greater need of social support may be least likely to get it. Second, most people have relatively little experience of dealing with others who are in the midst of a health crisis. For this reason, they may experience a great deal of uncertainty about what to say or do. Their anxiety may be heightened by the awareness that the victim is very vulnerable, and that inappropriate behaviour on support provider's part may aggravate the suffering of the person. Many times in such situations the support attempts become routine or ritualistic. Third, people generally hold a number of misconceptions about how people should react to their sickness. Beliefs about how much distress should be experienced and expressed and how long one should take in recovering, are some of the factors which are likely to influence the kind of support the family will provide. For example, family members may suspect that the patient is not doing enough if the recovery is not as expected within the stipulated time. Also, when expectations and beliefs are in contrast to what the sufferer holds, the attempt to provide support may prove counterproductive.

Indian families are intricately weaved into other subsystems of larger community network and cannot be seen in isolation. It is the prevailing cultural belief system which largely explains 'why do people fall sick, or suffer in general?' The Hindu cultural beliefs, for example, explain suffering of the victims in terms of their Karma's of previous lives. Family members and the patient frequently invoke principle of Karma to causally explain the chronic disease. This was quite evident in the study of the patients of tuberculosis and first heart attack (Agrawal & Dalal, 1993; Dalal & Singh, 1992). The finding was mixed regarding the association between belief in Karma and psychological recovery of the patient. This belief in some cases makes people fatalistic while in other cases optimistic about recovery. We still know little about the role of family beliefs in effective coping with the disease. Some chronic diseases and disabilities though stigmatizes the whole family, adversely affecting social prestige of the family and mar the marriage prospects of young family members (Dalal, 1994). For this reason, in cases of congenital and hereditary diseases, sometimes the attempt is to hide the disease or disability to save the family esteem and to avoid social humiliation. The patient suffers the perpetual anxiety of being rejected or being left out by the family members. Such anxiety was very much evident in cases of leprosy patients (Kushwah et al., 1981). Thus, family support not only fails to buffer them against the stresses of the disease, but may become an additional source of distress.

In brief, though the general finding that social and emotional support from the family is essential for effective coping with the disease, support does not always have intended consequences. The research which found evidence in favour has focused on short-term crisis, has taken normal families and has provided outsider's perspective. On the contrary, the findings about the support-failing have focused on long term crisis, have studied disturbed families and have looked at the internal family dynamics. There is a need for further research taking into consideration Indian value system and the disease context.

The Vulnerable Families

Research on family support has generally presumed family as an integrated and stable unit which puts up collective front to face a crisis. As Oommen (1991) puts it, this view of family from outside was perpetuated by the Indian researchers who happen to be mostly males from upper caste and urban middle class. It was easy for them to focus on the supportive aspects of family, that too from the recipient's perspective. It is no surprise that most of the evidence about the family support failing came from women studies and clinical work. These studies showed that an outwardly united and stable family could be crumbling from within. Change in socio-economic scenario and a change in social values, attitudes and expectations have further complicated the situation in which today there are very large number of families vulnerable to various stresses, and instead of being support providers, themselves need support. The factors which substantially contribute to family vulnerability are widespread poverty, unemployment, malnutrition, illiteracy and disease proneness in the society.

As it happens, many families have a history of high morbidity, greater susceptibility to infectious diseases and poor utilization of health-care services. In such high-risk families, presence of chronic illness of one family member may get linked with increased physical illness in other family members. Minuchin (1974) mentioned about psychosomatogenic families which are prone to physical illnesses due to environmental and psychological stresses, and easily get into a vicious family-illness cycle. In these cases, the family is not only responding to an illness in a maladaptive manner, but their methods of coping with the disease exacerbate and often precipitate illness episodes. Such families show the sign of acute strain, anger, depression, apathy and burn out while managing chronic family illness. In these instances, prolonged stress may not only destroy the role of family as a buffer for its members, but may destroy the family itself.

These vulnerable families could also be described in terms of socio-economic parameters. A number of such families are poverty stricken, lowly educated people living in urban slum areas. They are basically preoccupied with struggle for survival. Any additional crisis would greatly enhance the vulnerability of these families. The additional demands placed on scarce family resources could result in internal competition for scarce resources, mistrust, rivalry, jealousy and lack of communication. Then there are broken families, irrespective of their socio-economic status, where physical violence, verbal abuse and alcoholism are everyday occurrences. Quite often, such families have a long history of vulnerability, that is, have failed to cope with crises in the past. It is unlikely that such families could provide necessary support to its ailing members.

The above discussion should make it possible to develop some indicators to identify vulnerable families for the purpose of early intervention.

Based on the review of the available literature, it seems that the vulnerable families are characterized by:

1. *Social isolation:* Loss of meaningful contact with family networks, disease viewed as social stigma, chronic grief, feeling of shame and guilt
2. *Communication barrier:* Repression rather than expression of feelings, no sharing of worries and anxieties, conflicting perception of the disease and its causation
3. *Dysfunctional relationships:* Scapegoating for the crisis, physical and verbal abuse, lack of trust, displaced anger, negativism, over-indulgence or total indifference
4. *Rigidity:* Low adaptability to life changes, insulated to new information, overprotectiveness, exaggerated anxiety
5. *Family resources:* Inability to resolve family conflicts, inaction, no sense of personal control, burn out, high morbidity, family disintegration, withdrawal

Implications for Family Intervention

Family occupies the centre stage in Indian society and its significant role in providing support in crisis period of an individual can hardly be overemphasized. Despite the danger that the family support may fail, family as a unit is still the best bet for health-care intervention. The need is to strengthen the family's role as a caregiver in the changing world where the traditional bases of family functioning are eroding. Such efforts need to involve family networks, social and religious institutions, voluntary groups, family counsellors and researchers. The professionals can improve the situation by helping the patient and family members to develop realistic expectations about the problem and its ramifications, and also to have a shared understanding of the situation.

For any meaningful intervention, it is important to identify families which have the resilience and resources to provide support to its sick members, and the families which are vulnerable and need support. The mode of outside intervention in these two cases ought to be different. An early nearly identification of vulnerable families would be of much help in planning treatment procedures, secondary prevention or reha-bilitation of the people with chronic diseases. Larger family network and other social institutions could have a more active role in such instances. For this, it is necessary to have better dissemination of research findings and field experiences about the identification of vulnerable families and its effects on patient care.

The problem is that we still do not have much research base to sug-gest when the support efforts will not succeed even in the normal fami-lies. Work in the area of long-term health care is too scant to reach at some practical conclusions. It is not enough to know that family support works, but necessary to know which specific support efforts work in which set of conditions. A wide range of dispositional, cultural and contextual variables intervene between family support and coping responses. Research in this area deserves high priority to improve health status of the millions.

12

Folk Healing and Public Health-care Programmes

This chapter primarily focuses on meaning, tradition and practices of folk healing in India, the range of services they provide and their increasing popularity in the present times. The chapter examines scientific rationale of this indigenous medicinal knowledge and also discusses what makes them efficacious. The chapter explores the possibilities of integrating these practices within the existing public health-care programmes to provide holistic and comprehensive services to the patients suffering from chronic diseases.

The term healing has a Greek origin. The root term is 'healen', which implies physical and spiritual aspects of the human being to be rejuvenated. Chamber's Dictionary defines healing as 'becoming whole and healthy'. In a larger perspective, healing refers to treatment, recovery, well-being and restoration of physical and mental health. In the course of its ongoing struggle to cope with diseases, injuries and mental health problems, every society develops its own curative system based on its experiences. Folk healing is a collective and accumulated medicinal knowledge base of a society, which is rooted in experience and practical considerations. Folk healing finds its expression in proverbs, folklores, legends, poetry, rituals and mythologies. These sources tell us how life problems are created, construed and controlled by the collective efforts of the community. In its struggle to maintain harmony and order, every society attempts to develop ecologically valid understanding of human nature; its own theories of suffering and remedial measures (Kleinman, 1986). In many anthropological texts (e.g. Mariott, 1955), folk practices are considered within the little tradition, that is, the beliefs and practices of the masses. Shamans, spirits and local deities are all part of it. This is in contrast with the great tradition characterized by the practices based on classical and philosophical texts, like Vedas, Upanishads and the Gita. In this, God is held as the Supreme Self, realized through contemplative meditation and devotional worships. Indian system of medicine, in this sense, is part of the great tradition, with its own medicinal system, institutions, training programme and professional ethics. Folk medicine is part of the oral tradition with no texts and formal system. It is, however, a misconception that these two traditions are parallel and that the little tradition is subscribed by lower class and caste only (Mariott, 1955). In India, there has been a good deal of overlap between these two traditions, in terms of practices and clientele.

The folk systems, which evolved over more than four millennia, have weathered the vagaries of time, and have sustained (and thrived) in the present times on popular support. A wide range of healers and healing centres, which includes temples, *majars*, mosques, shrines, local deities, etc., are found in every nook and corner of the country. The burgeoning crowd that one sees around these places is a testimony to the fact that their relevance for healing the human psyche has not declined. Kakar (1982) has stated in his book, *Shamans, Mystics and Doctors* that India is a country of healers. There are shamans, gurus, *ojhas*, *tantriks*, priests and faith healers, who specialize in dealing with a variety of social and personal problems. The rapid progress in modern medicine has little affected the popularity of traditional systems. A gross estimate (VHAI, 1991) suggests that more than 90% of the Indian population believes and uses these services at some point in time. Nanda (2009) reported that faith in divine and spirituality has increased by 30% in the last five years. Thriving on folk wisdom and trusted by the masses, these folk healing practices are still an enigma for the health scientists.

The larger scientific community and modern medicine have remained critical and sceptical of the efficacy of these folk practices. These are held as pre-scientific and considered to be practiced by poor and tribal people (Kothari and Mehta, 1988). It is further argued that ignorance and backwardness are primarily responsible for adherence to these non-scientific practices. But, as Watts (1975) contended, traditional healing practices are called primitive, mystical and esoteric because our education does not prepare us to comprehend their sophistication. The works of Kakar (1982, 2003) and Kleinman (1980, 1988) have shown that most of these traditional practices are deeply entrenched in folk wisdom and sound theories of mind. They provide practical solutions to personal, familial and social problems, and have been integrated in the communal life. Despite their popular mass base, there is not enough work to test the premises of folk practices on the scientific crucible. There is a crying need to decipher folk healing and its knowledge base, and examine its import to augment therapeutic services. We need to develop methodologies and mindset to learn from this rich heritage to augment the existing public health-care system.

In India, the folk wisdom manifested in the traditional healing practices is, indeed, based on complex and cohesive systems of thoughts and beliefs, derived from philosophical texts and scriptures. Not only do the folk practices derive their legitimacy from the scriptures but they also proved to be effective vehicles to translate the essence of scriptures in dialects that a common man can follow. Folk beliefs and practices can be held as social representations of the formal texts and practical aspects of the classical theories. It is, however, a contentious issue how folk wisdom and scriptures complement each other, in which folk wisdom got distilled and documented in classical texts that in turn feed into the social life. In my view, folk and emancipatory (or scholarly) practices peacefully coexisted, though an undercurrent of mutual mistrust always remained. Of course, in the long history due to local influences, there are distortions, diversions and mutations in folk practices on the negative side, and improvisations, adaptations and innovations on the positive side. The folk systems have remained responsive to local needs and expectations.

We need to understand and acknowledge the contributions of these traditional practices in combating physical and mental illnesses we suffer from. Limited success of the biomedical model and modern psychotherapies, and their impersonal and market orientation has led to widespread discontentment (Foss, 2001; McFall, 2006). It is now widely accepted that psychotherapy works in the broader cultural context, which takes into consideration values and demands of the society (O'Hara, 2000). With the increase in stress-borne diseases and disorders, the spotlight is increasingly turning towards the age-old practices and examining their relevance in the modern world. There is a body of literature, which concurs the intuitive understanding that folk healers show about the working of human mind and its potential to alleviate suffering. The following section highlights the main features of these healing practices.

Main Features of Folk Healing Practices

Some of the important features that characterize most of the folk healing practices are presented here. Some of these characteristics of folk healing were discussed in other publications and presentations of the author (Dalal, 2011; Anand and Dalal, 2013).

Holistic Orientation

Local healers mostly focus on the overall condition of the person, rather than focusing on their disease condition only. Often the conjecture is that the disease condition is only a manifestation of unmanifested malaise, which needs to be looked into. Folk healing is holistic in the sense that they pay attention to the overall condition of the person. It takes body, mind, self and society within a framework of dynamic equilibrium. The holistic approach takes into consideration values, passions, beliefs, social interaction and spiritual orientation of a person in their healing practices.

The traditional healers often know intuitively about the close symbiotic relationship between the mind and the body—that the body cannot remain healthy when the mind is sick and vice versa. The healer creates conditions in which physiological processes are connected with meaning and relationships, so that our social world is linked recursively to one's inner experiences. In Ayurvedic tradition, which has greatly influenced the folk tradition in India, health is a balance among the body humours and the conditions of the external world mediated by diet and hierarchy of social relations organized around purity and pollution (Wujastyk, 1998).

Traditional healing focuses on the person, not on the problem. In healing sessions, the attention on the problem is only peripheral; the emphasis is on 'who is suffering?' These are the people, not the 'patients', who are helped to regain their normal functioning.

Thus, though some healing centres and healers specialize in the treatment of particular type of problems, often people with all kinds of crises frequent these places, be it physical or mental illness, family feuds, loss in business, marital discord or wrath of spirits. At healing centres, treatment for a wide range of problems does not vary significantly. At the Balaji temple in Ayodhya, for example, holy water is the standard treatment for all who come for solace.

Sacred Therapies

As stated by Kakar (1982), one of the distinguishing features of Indian healing practices is the role of the sacred. 'The whole weight of the community's religion, myths and history enters sacred therapy as the therapist proceeds to mobilize strong psychic energies inside and outside the patient ...' (p. 5). The sacred may be evoked in many forms, such as the local versions of Lord Shiva and Hanuman, spirits of ancestors, and demons. Different healing practices use different forms of sacred but for most of them the physical and metaphysical worlds overlap. Deities, demons and spirits are as much part of this physical world as they are of the metaphysical. Folk healing endeavours to preserve harmony between these two worlds.

The sacredness of the healing practices is further reinforced by the legends associated with the healer and/or healing centre. This author surveyed 18 such shrines in Uttar Pradesh and Rajasthan famous for their healing prowess. Each one of these centres had a story about how that shrine came into existence. It was either a deity who instructed a devotee in the dream, some paranormal phenomena observed on a particular spot, miraculous recovery near some enchanted grooves, deification of a sati, or boon bestowed on a devotee to have supernatural powers. These legends of derived powers are recounted with reverence by the visitors, who often know these healing stories by heart. There are rituals associated with these legends. For example, in many temples of mother goddess in eastern Uttar Pradesh, the devotees are expected to prostrate before the deity to offer their complete surrender. In the temple of a local deity in Chittor, Rajasthan, the patients are supposed to enter the temple crawling. The sacredness of these places is meticulously maintained by the priests, swamis, fakirs, *tantrik*s and gurus who manage these places. It may also be mentioned here that though sacred, many of these healing centres are secular and are frequented by the believers of different faiths and religion.

Healers as the Medium

Supernatural plays an important role in folk healing. In most of the folk practices, healers are mediators between the physical and the metaphysical. One can frequently find healers who are known for their ability to host a deity or spirit and under whose spell they acquire supernatural powers to control minds of the visitors and heal them. The healer becomes the medium through which others can communicate to deities and spirits. They get visions and can dispense with favours at will. As diviners they are presumed to be in direct communication with the supernatural and derive their healing powers through divine grace. They are both feared and revered by the local communities. Of course, they become diviners only on the occasions when possessed by some spirit. Otherwise, they are like any other commoner.

These traditional healers often belong to the same clan and subscribe to the same belief system. They are not formally educated to practice their art but learn it through apprenticeship and assisting their gurus. Quite often they inherit their right to practice and this remains a prerogative of few families whose members possess special powers to heal. No matter what is the background of the healer, they need long years of internal preparation to acquire a purity of body and mind. These healers are not supposed to charge for their services. In fact, it was widely believed that if they charge for their services their healing powers would go away. However, the community and patients are expected to compensate for their work by making them offerings. Most of the healers this author talked to also had some other sources of livelihood. They do farming, rear cattle, have small business or shop, or teach in a school. They offer a wide range of services, and are consulted on family and community matters. They are fortune tellers, medicine men, clairvoyagers and key informers about the community they serve. However, there seems to be a clear social hierarchy, which determines their status, power and mode of therapeutic relationship.

As observed by Kakar (2003), it is the matter of unquestioned faith in the paranormal powers of the healer, which is at the core of all positive outcomes. It is belief in the person in the healer, not his or her conceptual system or specific technique, which is of decisive importance in the healing process. What is of prime importance is the trust and confidence that a healer is capable of instilling in the minds of its clientele. The aura and authority of a healer is carefully cultivated through the stories of miraculous healing.

The tradition of guru as a healer is many times not consistent with the notion of a diviner. A good deal of healing takes place within the guru–disciple paradigm, the close relationship with the guru is an extension of the parent–child relationship (Kakar, 1991). Neki (1975) has discussed at length the therapeutic value of guru–*chela* relationship, and of surrender before the guru. The healing powers of guru were observed to reside in their ability to connect with the disciples' psyche, sending them the messages of strength and reassurance.

Socio-centric Treatment

Anonymity is rarely observed in the case of folk healing. In the folk tradition, any disease is a social event caused by a complex set of social, individual, supernatural and chance factors. Thus, a disease and its treatment are not personal or private affairs; it is a matter of concern for all. Social customs, traditions, moral strictures, interpersonal relations and supernatural are expected to play in causing various pathologies, as well as, in the treatment. Kleinman (1988) observed, in all Asian cultures body-self is not a secularized private domain of the individual person, but an organic part of the sacred, socio-centric world, a communication system involving exchange with others, including the divine. The person in these therapies is seen as embedded in a social hierarchy and in a network of relationships. One's family history, which includes ancestors also, is an important consideration in understanding the problem and deciding about the treatment modalities.

The healer and his/her healing practices are integral to the beliefs and practices of the local communities. The explanatory system, which a healer employs, is mostly congruous with the thinking of the masses. Evolved over centuries and verified in a countless number of cases, these beliefs about pain and suffering are compatible with the beliefs about life and supernatural. The theory of supernatural causation is widely believed and is frequently invoked to explain a wide range of happenings. Healing practices evolved around such beliefs thus have greater acceptability for its sick members.

It is a common observation that folk healing does not take place in the private chambers of the healers, but quite often it is a social activity held in an open place. People share their problems and consult the healer in full public view. Families and other community members also actively indulge in the treatment process. Everybody knows everyone's problem and it becomes a participatory venture to help out the suffering person.

Such an ethos is ideal for positive social construction of the problem and its remedy, which has the approval and acceptance of the community. These are the places where personal problem is no longer seen from the ego-centric perspective but within the larger social framework. Participation in social ritual and social nature of healing activities helps in relocating the person on a larger social canvas. This shift in focus from personal to social is important for relocating the ailing person within the social matrix.

Scientific Basis of Folk Therapies

Though medical science has serious questions regarding the efficacy of folk therapies, there is mounting empirical evidence that they heal. Surveys conducted in India show that more than 90% of the urban respondents believe in the efficacy of folk therapies in the treatment of physical and mental illnesses (Purohit, 2002). This popularity of folk practices is not due to the socio-cultural beliefs, which people have but due to their observed efficacy in a variety of situations. It is no surprise that the faith in the efficacy of folk practices have survived in the long history, with all advances in modern medicine.

The work of Kleinman (1988) and others have also shown that such beliefs in the efficacy of folk therapies is not just the matter of faith but are also supported by medical research. However, in such scientific testing there are always problems of finding proper methodologies to verify the efficacy healing outcomes. Often such positive outcomes of folk healing are attributed to placebo effect and dismissed as unexplainable. Because of the lack of methodologies, there is a real dearth of studies that can throw light on the process and mechanism underlying such healing.

In this section, on the basis of available literature and evidences an attempt will be made to demystify the healing process. If we understand how these traditional practices work, it should be possible to derive some insights into modern psychotherapies.

One factor that renders conjectures hazardous is that these folk therapies differ in terms of their sophistication and specialization. The cultural diversity of India has facilitated the growth of diverse systems in different regions of the country. It is a daunting task for any social scientist to capture the range and diversity of these healing practices. As Kiev (1965) has noted, differentiation in the therapeutic practices are contingent on the civilizational advancement of a particular society. In a tribal society, as among the Bhils in south Rajasthan, the healer is medicine man, village elder and a consultant on all important matters, besides being a holy man, whereas in arid but more prosperous zones of Jodhpur and Jaisalmer, the *bhopas* specialize in the treatment of different species of snakes and snake biting.

As discussed elsewhere (Anand, 2011; Dalal, 2001), traditional healing practices primarily deal with psychological aspects of the problem. No matter what are the actual causes of the problem, be it organic, emotional or social, the suffering is viewed as a state of mind, a subjective experience. Healers develop their own psychological theories about the functioning of human mind, which are implicit in their healing practices. Kakar (1982, 2003) has concluded on the basis of an in-depth analysis of the traditional healing systems in India and that the healing powers reside primarily within the patient's mind rather than in the tenets of various faiths and ideologies. It is the tremendous outpouring and channelizing of a patient's emotions and faith, rather than any specific aspects of healer's personality or methods, which seem to be responsible for the dramatic cures. Similar observations were made by clinical psychologists Frank and Frank (1991) about western psychotherapies as well, 'The apparent success of healing methods based on different or incompatible ideologies and methods compels the conclusion that the healing power resides in the patient's state of mind, not in the validity of a particular theoretical scheme or technique' (p. 111). More recently, an extensive empirical study confirmed this finding

(Anand, 2011). Healing is, thus a by-product of the interaction between the healer and the person, particularly the way subliminal messages are received and interpreted.

While discussing these folk healing practices, it should be clear that all such healing experiences are not emancipatory, nor do they lead to elimination of the problem. Practice of Yoga and meditation may lead to liberating experience and may give insight into the ephemeral nature of worldly problems. Traditional therapies, on the other hand, focus on the changing unhealthy patterns of thinking, feeling and behaving, and prepare the person to face the vicissitudes of the problems in their social world. At times, the actual problem may not go away but as a consequence of the traditional therapy people learn to live with it. These therapies soothe the troubled ego of the person. In other words, the therapy may result in (i) symptom relief and (ii) improved functioning. Symptom relief is achieved by lowering expectations, whereas improved functioning is contingent on remodelled pattern of social interaction, for which others in the family have to change as well.

It may be convincingly conjectured that folk practitioners know intuitively what works in the healing sessions. Their training and conceptual tools, however, may lead to different interpretations and articulations of the process than what a health psychologist would construe. In this section, attempt is made to unravel the healing process in traditional practices from a social-psychological perspective.

The Faith That Heals

In the beginning of the last century, William Osler (1910), the founding father of modern medicine, wrote an article 'The Faith that Heals'. In this, he extolled the important role of faith in health, healing and medicine (Osler, 1910). He argued, 'Faith is indeed one of the miracles of human nature, which science is as ready to accept as it is to study its marvellous effects' (p. 1470). Osler asserted that the impact of faith is very real and cannot be denied. Sixty-five years later, Jerome Frank (1975) revisited this theme and wrote a paper by the same title. Frank agreed with Osler but lamented, '(faith) is an important topic that is conspicuously absent from the medical school curriculum' (p. 127). Cassel (1991) found no evidence of 'faith' being part of medical curriculum. In recent years, there is increasing evidence that medical science is getting interested in study-ing the positive role of faith in the face of mounting clinical evidence (Levin, 2009). Research in the areas of hope, learned optimism, positive illusion and psycho-neuroimmunology have found repeated evidences of the healing powers of faith.

Faith healing does not imply faith in supernatural or paranormal phenomena and their role in the recovery of the person. It is not impor-tant in whom you have faith—God, doctor, self, family or other agency. The empirical finding is overwhelming that faith heals, stronger the faith better the healing is. Though in science an empirical finding is not a sufficient precondition, unless these findings can be weaved into a plausible theory to explain the phenomenon. This is still a challenge for medical science where, oftentimes, terms like faith and healing arouse negative reactions.

Burgeoning crowd at the traditional healing centres, particularly on the auspicious days, is a clear testimony of their popularity and healing prowess. Kakar (1982, 2003) has evinced that faith builds hope, positive construction, initiative, and a host of other positive emotions necessary for healing to take place. As argued by Kakar, such positive thinking and feelings at healing centres is infectious and create an atmosphere of possibilities and miraculous healing.

Subliminal Healing Messages

Healing is primarily in the transaction that takes place between the healer and the suffering individual. Whatever be the nature of problem people suffer from, they experience emotional distress and manifest psychological symptoms of anxiety, fear, withdrawal, dissociation, etc. These symptoms impair their physical and mental functioning, making their suffering worse. An experienced healer knows that these people need reassurance. A healer creates an aura of authority over the natural and supernatural, and reinforces the belief of a sufferer and his or her family that he can control the course of events. For this, it is not very important what kind of verbal exchange takes place between the two, but how effectively the non-verbal messages are put across and received. The healing rituals make extensive use of cultural symbolism to send the healing messages across. The messages that are subliminally transmitted, and not mediated by the conscious mind are more effective in reassuring the person that the things are likely to improve.

It is not clearly known how such subliminal messages are exchanged. These messages are communicated through cultural symbols, legends and myths, which arouse positive emotions that heal. These may have a powerful influence on the person, as their effect is accentuated by an aura created by the healer. These messages are received and processed by the unconscious mind. In an article published in the *Lancet*, Evans and Richardson (1988) have shown that positive suggestions to the anaesthetized patient in the operating room lead to not only less discomfort after surgery but also to early discharge from the hospital. There is much work to suggest that subliminal messages bring change in attitudes and emotions. Such cassettes and audiotapes with subliminal messages are frequently available in the market, which claim to facilitate self-healing (Galbraith and Barton, 1990). Lipton (2008) in his recent book *Biology of Beliefs* has discussed power of the unconscious mind, arguing that 'Eighty percent of the effect of antidepressants, as measured in clinical trials, could be attributed to the placebo effect' (p. 110), which demonstrates the power of subconscious mind.

Broadening the Domain of Experience

Folk healing aims to bring out the person from the narrow, myopic view of the problem and help them experience the larger social and metaphysical reality. The healing process connects people with their past and future, with living and dead, with demon and divine to broaden their range of life experience. Various rituals and ceremonies solicit the indulgence of ancestors and departed relations, who are held as part of the wider support group. People develop a sense of belonging to a larger cross-section of people and learn to situate their problem in the larger social matrix.

Healing thus facilitates the process of becoming social being from an individual being in the face of a crisis. Healing centres are the places of intense social activities where people learn to deal with the problem in newer ways. The crises experience becomes an opportunity to fully integrate the person into the social mainstream. Imposition of social meaning on one's illness and exposure to cultural symbolism brings the person face to face with others in the society and participation in the healing rituals implies that the person is accepted as equals by those who matter in the community. Healing occurs through broadening of the network of relationships (Kapoor, 2003). Community healing marks the transition of a person from a personal to social identity. People develop a feeling of responsibility, competence and interdependence; and feel reassured that they are not alone, nor their predicament is unique.

Repatterning of Affective Responses

All healers know from experience that emotions could be destructive and once emotions follow a predictable self-damaging path, suffering can be endemic. Folk healing thus endeavours to break this pattern of emotions. Repatterning of affective responses may follow different tracks. One is, redefining of relationship with self, family and social network from very personal to role-specific; from spontaneous to functional mode of affective relationships. Another is changing from idiosyncratic conflicts and defences to conventional conflicts and ritualized symptoms. In doing so, they develop a sense of sharing and togetherness. Often shamans provide a kind of corrective emotional experience that leads to repatterning of defences without real curative insights.

Most of the healing encounters are of affective nature. These encounters make people realize their vulnerabilities and openly vent out their feelings. Siegel (1991) observed in his vast clinical experience that when you put your feelings outside, you heal inside. Anger, anxiety, depression, fear and many other feelings are unhealthy only if they remain buried inside, unexpressed and not dealt with. When one goes beyond one's surface emotions and begins to acknowledge one's real fears, one can break through the resentments and disappointments one holds, and herein begins the process of true healing (Anand, 2004, 2011). In the healing process, people not only experience new emotions that change their way of experiencing the tragic happenings. Such repatterning of emotions is often followed by a new pattern in social relationships. Change in emotions thus lead to a more adaptive behavioural sequel, and show social maturity to handle social and moral demands.

Creating Healthy Imageries

The success of any healing centre lies in creating strong imageries of health, well-being and prosperity. Through aroma, chanting, drumming and symbols, an ambience is created conducive to the arousal of some familiar imagery associated with strength and security. Stories of miraculous recovery from a disease or disability are told and retold to sustain imageries of hope and optimism. These imageries are often not of the kind as found in yoga and meditation, but relate to the mundane world and its objects. Many safe and effective techniques are evolved and intricately integrated in the healing rituals to arouse cultural imageries of well-being. Such imageries are powerful tools to bring about desired change in attitudes and expectations from healing encounters.

That imageries bring physiological changes need no hard evidence. The very image of a ripe mango can wet one's mouth. The impact of imageries (or imagination) on physiological processes as varied as respiration, blood pressure, heart rate, muscle tension, bowel movement, salivation, etc., is common experience for any one. Imageries can bring major changes in the functioning of autonomic nervous system. In recent times, visualization is used as a powerful tool in the treatment of varied diseases, even cancer (Sheikh et al., 1989).

The traditional healers master the art of heightening people's suggestibility to induce particular type of imageries and healing messages. During healing sessions, *bhopa*s of Rajasthan beat the drums and everyone joins in a circular two-stepped hoping dance. The rhythm of the drum and steps in the dance synchronize and create a kinaesthetic experience for both the *bhopa*s and their believers. This was presumed to invoke the spirit of benevolent ancestors who can bestow health and happiness. There are many other techniques used by the folk practitioners to alter states of mind, such as chanting, slow breathing, rhythmic dancing, fasting, sensory and social isolation. This facilitated lulling of the conscious mind, rendering the unconscious mind more receptive to positive imageries induced by the healer. The other ways of creating desired imageries and mindset is through getting into a trance-like state. The healers in many parts of the country get into an altered state of consciousness through elaborate preparation and rituals, when they are supposed to be possessed by some divine spirit. In that state, the shamans and healers are presumed to be in direct communication with other deities, demons, spirits and gods. They exhibit bizarre but familiar behaviour, which has symbolic meaning, transporting the audience in a world of paranormal visions and experiences. How these techniques actually work is still an enigma to the scientific community.

Building Positive Social Ethos

Most of the traditional healers know from their personal experience that treating the person is not enough. Unless the family and the community to which the person belongs change, any improvement in their mental health will be short-lived. Very often, the problem for which people come to a healer has its genesis in unhealthy social relationships. It is therefore imperative that all concerned parties participate in the healing process.

In the case of hysterical outbursts, as we observed at one healing centre, what is gratifying for the women was that suddenly the whole family had woken up to her existence and were concerned about her needs and welfare. Many women reported that after their recovery no one in the family was ill-treating her for the fear of Balaji (the monkey god). The family and other relatives who participate in the healing rituals, many of which take place in the home setting, are directed to bring about attitudinal change. Most of these activities are not systematically planned by the healer.

Take the example of parents of children having a major disease or disability suffer silently and need reassurance that things will improve. The Avari Mata temple in south Rajasthan is flourishing for the last four decades as a healing centre for polio and paralysis. The suddenness of the attack and incapacitation of the patient makes the family scared and confused. Taking it as a wrath of the mother goddess and finding medical treatment ineffective, many of them are rushed to this temple when struck by the disease. Situated in a hilly terrain with a quiet river flowing along, this place is an ideal location for outing. The patients who arrive with family members camp here for several days. On my visit to that place, I found a party atmosphere all around, where people sitting in small groups were chatting, singing bhajans or feasting on the riverside. With so much sharing and exchange of information, their fears and anxieties had already taken a back seat. They knew they are not alone in that tragic predicament and that there are people who are worse than them. There was an air of expectancy about the recovery; many stories of miraculous healing were already doing their rounds. All this not only helps in overcoming the initial shock but also creates a mental state conducive to physical recovery.

Folk Healing and Public Health Programmes

India has a large network of public health-care system. Primary health care is provided through a network of sub-centres, primary health-care centres, community health centres and district hospitals. In rural areas, most primary health care is provided either by sub-centres or primary health-care centres, whereas in urban areas it is provided via health clinics and hospitals. Primary health care included maternal and child care, including family planning, immunization against major infectious diseases, prevention and control of locally endemic diseases, appropriate treatment of common diseases and injuries, provision of essential drugs, education concerning prevailing health problems and ways to deal with them, provision of adequate food and nutrition and adequate supply of clean water. Government health policy of primary health care through primary health centres (PHCs) were framed along WHO guideline following Alma-Ata Declaration of 1978. Medical doctors and paramedical staff manage these PHCs.

Folk healers with some training can easily manage many of the activities of PHC. They have been almost ignored by the vast network of these PHCs and excluded from health programmes. In India, these folk healers have been providing services for the whole range of organic and mental health problems to all sections of the society for the last four millennia. The efficacy of folk healing is doubted by health professionals, scientists and rationalists. Folk healers are often called quacks, or their efficacy is attributed to placebo effect. Critics of western psychotherapies and of biomedicine have also not ruled out placebo effect behind claims of the success of the medical therapies. Erwin (1959) emphatically argued with supportive evidences that about 65–70% improve after treatment regardless of the type of treatment. Kiev (1965) and Frank (1974) also reported similar findings. In recent times, *APA Monitor* prominently featured a research study that showed that the active ingredient in the treatment of 225 depressed people was the clients' active participation, and strength and duration of therapeutic bond between the therapist and the client (*APA Monitor*, September 1996). Wampold (2001) has shown in an extensive survey that what is of prime importance in psychotherapy is psychotherapist as a person whom the client can trust, not his method or training.

Modern medicine has not fulfilled the expectations it has aroused at the initial stage. Adherence to this model has helped in reducing mortality and enhancing life expectancy, though at the cost of poor quality of physical health, with an increasingly large population suffering from chronic diseases. As Lown (2007) has observed,

> At a time when doctors are performing the near miracles, the profession's reputation is increasingly discredited. More and more, patients complain about not being listened to and being abandoned. As medicine has conquered acute illness, it increasingly fails in coping with the growing toll of chronic disease—arthritis, cardiovascular ailments, cancer, diabetes, pulmonary impairments and neurological derangements. Lacking a cure, these illnesses require the art of healing for which the contemporary physician is poorly trained. (p. 12)

Modern health-care services are in crisis today; and serious questions are raised about their efficacy in managing the challenge of health and illness in present times. The discontentment is evident from the fact that more than one-third of their clientele in the west is now turning towards alternative therapies, not covered by their insurance policies. Modern psychotherapies are going through a crisis of identity and a debate is raging about their goals, philosophy and moral vision (VandenBos, 1996; McFall, 2006). There is renewed interest in religion and spirituality and their role in therapeutic process (Miller and Thoresen, 2003). Traditional healing therapies of India have much to contribute to this end. The rich know-how and techniques employed in traditional therapies to bring about attitude change can provide new insights to evolve more relevant and efficient health care.

Dalal and Misra (2006) proposed a comprehensive health-care model to incorporate the various facets of health and well-being and to benefit from the traditional health-care systems. In this model, health is seen along three main domains, that is, *restoration, maintenance* and *growth*.

Restoration refers to bringing the person back from the state of illness to the state of health; *maintenance* refers to taking preventing measures and keeping good health; *growth* refers to improving quality of one's health, that is, psycho-spiritual health. Defining health in this holistic manner carves roles for medical professionals, practitioners of alternative medicine and folk healers. Health-care programmes can be efficacious if a place can be created for these local healers in the endeavour to provide better quality services.

References

Abramson, L.Y., Seligman, M.E.P. & Teasdale, J. (1978). Learned helplessness in humans: Critique and reformulation. *Journal of Abnormal Psychology, 87,* 49–74.

Affleck, G., Allen, D.G., Tennen, H., McGrade, B.J. & Ratzan, S. (1985). Causal and control cognitions in parents' coping with chronically ill children. *Journal of Social and Clinical Psychology, 2,* 367–77.

Affleck, G., Tennen, H., Pfeiffer, C. & Fifield, J. (1987). Appraisals of control and predictability in adapting to a chronic disease. *Journal of Personality and Social Psychology, 53,* 273–279.

Agrawal, M. & Dalal, A.K. (1993). Beliefs about the world and recovery from myocardial infarction. *Journal of Social Psychology, 133*(3), 385–394.

Agarwal, M., Dalal, A.K., Agarwal, D.K. & Agarwal, R.K. (1994). Positive life orientation and recovery from myocardial infraction. *Social Science and Medicine, 38,* 152–160.

Agarwal, M. & Naidu, R.K. (1988). Impact of desirable and undesirable life events on health. *Journal of Personality and Clinical Studies, 4,* 53–62.

Almeida, D.M. (2005). Resilience and vulnerability to daily stressors assessed via diary methods. *Current Directions in Psychological Science, 14,* 64–68.

Anand, J. (2004). Working through emotional pain: A narrative study of healing process. *Psychological Studies, 49,* 185–192.

———. (2011). *Healing Narratives of Women: A Psychological Perspective.* Jaipur, India: Rawat.

Anand, J. & Dalal, A.K. (2013). Concept, characteristics and process of psychological healing. In G. Misra (Ed.), *History of Science, Philosophy and Culture: Psychology and Psychoanalysis,* vol. 9 (pp. 697–710). New Delhi: Centre for Studies in Civilizations.

Antelius., E. (2009). Whose body is it anyway? Verbalization, embodiment, and the creation of narratives. *Health, 13,* 361–379.

Antonovsky, A. (1987). *Unraveling the Mystery of Health: How People Manage Stress and Stay Well.* San Francisco: Jossey-Bass Publishers.

———. (1988). *Unravelling the Mystery of Health: How People Manage Stress and Stay Well.* London: Jossey-Bass.

Averill, J.R. (1973). Personal control over aversive stimuli and its relationship to stress. *Psychological Bulletin, 80,* 145–157.

Balfour, G. (1999). *How qualitative researchers manage ethical dilemmas: Investigating the connections between ethics and theory*. Paper presented at the first annual Conference on Advances in Qualitative Research Method, Edmonton, Alberta, Canada, February.

Bandura, A. (1977). Self efficacy: Toward a unifying theory of behavioural change. *Psychological Review, 84*(2), 191–215.

Banerjee, A. & Sanyal, D. (2012). Dynamics of doctor-patient relationship: A cross-sectional study on concordance, trust, and patient enablement. *Journal of Family and Community Medicine, 19*(1), 12–19.

Banerjee, D. (1986). *Social Service and Health Service Development in India: Sociology of Formation of an Alternative Paradigm*. New Delhi: Lok Paksha.

———. (1993). Simplistic approach to health policy analysis. *Economic and Political Weekly, 12*(June), 1207–1210.

Bard, M. & Dyk, R.B. (1956). The psychodynamic significance of beliefs regarding the cause of serious illness. *Psychoanalytic Review, 43*, 146–162.

Bar-On, D. (1984). Causal attributions and rehabilitation of heart attack patients. *Psychosomatic Medicine, 46*, 23–37.

Basu, J. (1995). Gender stereotype, self-ideal disparity, and neuroticism in Bengali families. *Indian Journal of Social Work, 56*, 298–311.

Baumeister, R.F. & Newman, L.S. (1994). How stories make sense of personal experiences: Motives that shape autobiographical narratives. *Personality and Social Psychology Bulletin, 20*, 676–690.

Becker, M.H. & Maiman, L.A. (1975). Sociobehavioural determinants of compliance with health and medical care recommendations. *Medical Care, 13*, 10–24.

Becker, M.H., Maiman, L.A., Kirscht, J.P., Huefner, D.P. & Drachman, R.H. (1977). The health belief model and dietary compliance: A field experiment. *Journal of Health and Social Behaviour, 18*, 348–366.

Beecher, H.K. (1955). The powerful placebo. *Journal of American Medical Association, 159*, 1602–1606.

Benedetti, F. (2011). Many placebo effects. *Spanda Journal, 2*(1), 5–8.

Benham, M.K.P. (2007). Mo'Olelo: On culturally relevant story making from an indigenous perspective. In D.J. Claindinin (Ed.), *Handbook of Narrative Inquiry: Mapping a Methodology* (pp. 512–534). Thousand Oaks, CA: SAGE Publications.

Benson, H. (1997). *Timeless Healing: The Power and Biology of Beliefs*. New York: Simon & Schuster.

Bergner, M., Bobbitt, R.A., Carter, W.B. & Gilson, B.S. (1981). The sickness impact profile: Development and final revision of a health status measure. *Medical Care, 19*, 787–805.

Bergner, M., Bobbitt, R.A., Kressel, S., Pollard, W.E., Gilson, B.S. & Morris, J.R. (1976). The Sickness Impact Profile: Conceptual formulation and methodology for the development of a health status measure. *International Journal of Health Services, 6*, 393–415.

Bergvik, S. (2008). *Psychological factors in the recovery of coronary artery disease patient in northern Norvey.* Unpublished doctoral dissertation, University of Tromso, Norvey.

Berkman, L.F. & Syme, S.L. (1979). Social network, host resistance and mortality: A nine-year follow-up study of Alameda county residents. *American Journal of Epidemiology, 109,* 186–204.

Bharat, S. (1991). Research on family structure and problems: Review, implications and suggestions. In Unit for Family Studies (Ed.), *Research on Families with Problems in India.* Bombay: Tata Institute of Social Sciences Publication.

Bhattacharyya, D. (2001). The effect of Type-A behavior and locus of control in the coping styles: A study of coronary heart disease patients. *Indian Journal of Clinical Psychology, 28*(2), 181–184.

Bhawuk, D.P.S. (2012). *Spirituality and Indian Psychology: Lessons from the Bhagavad Gita.* New York: Springer.

Blazer, D.G. (1982). Social support and mortality in an elderly community population. *American Journal of Epidemiology, 115,* 684–694.

Borne, H.W., Pruyn, J.F.A. & Mey, K.D. (1986). Self-help in cancer patients: A review of studies on the effects of contacts between fellow-patients. *Patient Education and Counseling, 8,* 367–385.

Braun, V. & Clark, V. (2006). Using thematic analysis in psychology, *Qualitative Research in Psychology, 3,* 77–101.

Brehm, J.W. (1966). *A theory of Psychological Reactance.* New York: Academic Press.

Brehm, S.S. & Brehm, J.W. (1981). *Psychological Reactance: A Theory of Freedom and Control.* New York: Academic Press.

Brewin, C.R. (1984). Perceived controllability of life-events and willingness to prescribe psychotropic drugs. *British Journal of Social Psychology, 23,* 285–287.

Brickman, P., Rabinowitz, V.C., Karuza, J., Coates, D., Cohn, E. & Kidder, L. (1982). Models of helping and coping. *American Psychologist, 37,* 368–384.

Broyard, A. (1992). *Intoxicated by My Illness and Other Writings on Life and Death.* New York: Ballantine Books.

Bruner, J.S. (1986). *Actual Minds, Possible Worlds.* Cambridge: Harvard University Press.

Bulman, R.J. & Wortman, C.B. (1977). Attributions of blame and coping in the 'real world': Severe accident victims react to their lot. *Journal of Personality and Social Psychology, 35,* 351–363.

Burish, T.C. & Bradley, L.A. (1983). *Coping with Chronic Disease: Research and Applications.* New York: Academic Press.

Cameron, K.S. & Caza, A. (2004). Contributions to the discipline of positive organizational scholarship. *American Behavioral Scientist, 47*(6), 731–739.

Caplan, G. (1974). *Support System and Community Mental Health.* New York: Behavioural Publications.

Caplan, R.D. (1979). Social support, person-environment fit and loving. In L.A. Ferman & J.P. Gordus (Eds), *Mental Health and Economy.* Kalamazoo: Upjahn Institute.

Caplan, R.D., Naidu, R.K. & Tripathi, R.C. (1986). Accepting advice: A modifier of how social support affects well-being. *Journal of Personal and Social Relationships, 3,* 213–228.

Capra, F. (1982). *The Turning Point: Science, Society and the Rising Culture.* London: Flamingo Books.

Carstairs, G.M. (1957). *The Twice Born.* London: Hogarth Press.

Carstairs, G.M. & Kapur, R.L. (1976). *The Great Universe of Kota: Stress Change and Mental Disorder in an Indian Village.* London: Hogarth Press.

Carver, C.S., Harris, S.D., Lehman, J.M., Dural, L.A., Antoni, M.H., et al. (2000). How important is the perception of perceived control? Studies of early stage breast cancer patients. *Personality and Social Psychology Bulletin, 26,* 139–149.

Cashin, A., Browne, G., Bradbury, J. & Mulder, A.M. (2013). The effectiveness of narrative therapy with young people with autism. *Journal of Child and Adolescent Mental Health Nursing, 26*(1), 32–41.

Cassel, J. (1976). The contribution of the social environment to host resistance. *Journal of Epidemiology, 104,* 107–123.

Cassell, E.J. (1991). *The Nature of Suffering and the Goals of Medicine.* New York: Oxford University Press.

Chadda, R.K. & Deb, K.S. (2013). Indian family systems, collectivistic society and psychotherapy. *Indian Journal of Psychiatry, 55*(6), 299–319.

Chambliss, C. & Murray, E.J. (1979). Cognitive Procedures for smoking reduction: Symptom versus efficacy attribution. *Cognitive Therapy and Research, 3,* 91–95.

Channa, Subhadra Mitra (1997). Gender and social space in a Haryana village. *Indian Journal of Gender Studies, 1,* 21–34.

———. (1996). Personal vulnerability and interpretive authority in narrative research. In R. Josselson (Ed.), *The Narrative Story of Lives: Vol. 4. Ethics and Process in Narrative Study of Lives* (pp. 45–59). Thousand Oaks, CA: SAGE Publications.

———. (2011). Narrative inquiry: Still a field in the making. In N.K. Denzin & Y.S. Lincoln (Eds), *The SAGE Handbook of Qualitative Research* (4th ed., pp. 421–434). Los Angeles: SAGE Publications.

Chatterji, S.A. (1997). *The Indian Women's Search for an Identity.* New Delhi: Vikas Publishing House.

Clegg, F. (1988). Bereavement. In S. Fisher & J. Reasdon (Eds), *Handbook of Life Stress, Cognition and Health.* New York: John Wiley.

Cobb, S. (1976). Social support as a moderator of life stress. *Psychosomatic Medicine, 37,* 300–314 .

———. (1979). Social support and health through the life course. In R.M. White (Ed.), *Aging from Birth to Death: Interdisciplinary Perspectives.* Boulder: Westview Press.

Cohen, F. & Lazarus, R.S. (1979). Coping with the stresses of illness. In G.C. Stone, F. Cohen & N.E. Adler (Eds), *Health Psychology: A Handbook.* San Francisco: Jossey-Bass.

Cohen, S. (2005). Keynote presentation at the eighth International Congress of Behavioral Medicine: The Pittsburgh common cold studies: Psychosocial predictors of susceptibility to respiratory infectious illness. *International Journal Behavioural Medicine, 12*, 123–131.

Colletti, G. & Kopel, S.A. (1979). Maintaining behavior changes: An investigation of three maintenance strategies and the relationship of self-attribution to the long-term reduction of cigarette smoking. *Journal of Consulting and Clinical Psychology, 47*, 614–617.

Collins, B.E., Martin, J.C., Ashmore, R.D. & Ross, L. (1973). Some dimensions of the internal—external metaphor in theories of personality. *Journal of Personality, 41*, 471–492.

Cousins, N. (1979). *Anatomy of an Illness.* New York: Norton.

Coyne, J.C. & DeLongis, A. (1986). Going beyond social support: The role of social relationships in adaptation. *Journal of Consulting and Clinical Psychology, 54*, 454–464.

Coyne, J.C., Wortman, C.B. & Lehman, D.R. (1988). The other side of support: Emotional over involvement and miscarried helping. In B.H. Gottfield (Ed.), *Marshaling Social Support: Formats, Processes, and Effects.* Newbury Park, CA: SAGE Publications.

Crano, W.D. & Prislin, R. (2006). Attitude and persuasion. *Annual Review of Psychology, 57*, 345–347.

Cromwell, R.L., Butterfleld, E.C., Brayfield, F.M. & Curry, J.J. (1977). *Acute Myocardial Infarction: Reaction and Recovery.* St. Louis: Mosby.

Dalal, A.K. (1988). Reactions to tragic life events: An attributional model of psychological recovery. In A.K. Dalal (Ed.), *Attribution Theory and Research.* New Delhi: Wiley Eastern.

———. (1994). *Family attitudes and beliefs in community rehabilitation practices.* Paper presented at the UN Conference on 'Stronger Family-Stronger Children' Victoria, Canada.

———. (1999). Health beliefs and coping with a chronic illness. In G. Misra (Ed.), *Psychological Perspectives on Stress and Health* (pp. 100–125). New Delhi: Concept Publishers.

———. (2000). Living with a chronic disease: Healing and psychological adjustment in Indian society. *Psychology and Developing Societies, 12*(1), 67–82.

———. (2001). Health psychology. In J. Pandey (Ed.), *Psychology in India Revisited: Development in the Discipline* (pp. 356–411). New Delhi: SAGE Publications.

———. (2005). Integrating traditional health care systems with modern medicine. *Journal of Health Management, 7*(2), 249–262.

———. (2010). *Indigenous belief system and its consequences for mental and physical health practices.* In Souvenir and Abstracts, 36th National Annual Conference of the Indian Association of Clinical Psychology (1–3 February 2010) held at NIMHANS, Bangalore.

———. (2011). Folk wisdom and traditional healing practices: Some lessons for modern psychotherapies. In M. Cornelisson, G. Misra & S. Verma (Eds), *Foundations of Indian Psychology* (pp. 21–35). New Delhi: Pearson.

Dalal, A.K. (2013). Salience of indigenous healing practices for health care planning in India. In R.C. Tripathi & Y. Sinha (Eds), *Psychology as a Policy Science* (pp. 193–210). New Delhi: Springer.

Dalal, A.K. & Agarwal, R. (1987). Causal thinking and expectation of success in the achievement context. *Journal of General Psychology, 114,* 57–68.

Dalal, A.K. & Pande, N. (1988). Psychological recovery of accident victims with temporary and permanent disability. *International Journal of Psychology, 23,* 25–40.

Dalal, A.K. & Sethi, A. (1988). An attributional study of high and low need achievers in India. *Journal of Social Psychology, 128*(1), 55–64.

Dalal, A.K. & Singh, A.K. (1992). Role of causal and recovery beliefs in the psychological adjustment to a chronic disease. *Psychology and Health, 6,* 193–203.

Dalal, A.K. & Tripathi, M. (1987). When the help is denied: A study of attribution linked affective reactions. *International Journal of Psychology, 22,* 1–15.

Dalal, A.K. & Weiner, B. (1988). Measurement of causal stability and prediction of expectancy of success. In A.K. Dalal (Ed.), *Attribution Theory and Research.* New Delhi: Wiley Eastern.

Davar, B. (1998). *Mental Health of Indian Women: A Feminist Agenda.* New Delhi: SAGE Publications.

Davidsen, A.S. & Reventlow, S. (2010). 'It takes some time to get into the rhythm— and to slow the flow of thought': A qualitative study about experience of time and narrative in psychological interventions in general practice. *Health, 14,* 348–368.

Dembo, T., Leviton, G.L. & Wright, B.A. (1956). Adjustment to misfortune: A problem of social Psychological rehabilitation. *Artificial Limbs, 3*(2), 4–62.

Denollet, J. (2000). Type D personality: A potential factor redefined. *Journal of Psychosomatic Research, 49*(4), 255–266.

———. (2004). Type D personality in perspective. *Journal of Psychosomatic Research, 56,* 584–596.

Derogatis, L.R. (1977). *Psychological Adjustment to Illness Scale.* Baltimore: Clinical Psychometric Research.

Derogatis, L.R. (1991). Personality, stress, disease and bias in epidemiological research. *Psychological Inquiry, 2,* 238–242.

Dweck, C.S. (1975). The role of expectations and attributions in the alleviation of learned helplessness. *Journal of Personality and Social Psychology, 31,* 675–685.

Edvardsson, D., Rasmussen, B.H. & Riessman, C.K. (2003). Ward atmospheres of horror and healing: A comparative analysis of narrative. *Health, 7*(4), 377–396.

Emons, W.H., Mols, F., Pelle, A.J.M., Smolderen, K.G. & Denollet, J. (2012). Type D assessment in patients with chronic heart failure and peripheral arterial disease: Evaluation of the experimental DS (3) scale using item response theory. *Journal of Personality Assessment, 94,* 210–219.

Engel, G.L. (1977). The need for a new medical model: A challenge for biomedicine. *Science, 196,* 129–136.

Evans, C. & Richardson, P.H. (1988). Improved recovery and reduced post-operative stay after therapeutic suggestions during general anesthesia. *Lancet, 332*(27 August), 491–492.

Fazio, R.H. & Olson, M.A. (2002). Implicit measures in social cognition research: Their meaning and use. *Annual Review of Psychology, 54*, 297–327.

Felton, B.J. & Revenson, T.A. (1984). Coping with chronic illness: A study of illness controllability and the influence of coping strategies on psychological adjustment. *Journal of Consulting and Clinical Psychology, 52*, 343–353.

Fielding, J.W., Fagg, S.L., Jones, B.G., et al. (1983). An interim report of a prospective, randomized, controlled study of adjuvant chemotherapy in operable gastric cancer: British stomach Cancer Group. *World Journal of Surgery, 7*, 390–399.

Fife, B.L. (1994). The conceptualization of meaning in illness. *Qualitative Health Research, 9*(6), 786–802.

Ford, S., Fallowfield, L. & Lewis, S. (1996). Doctor-patient interactions in oncology. *Social Science and Medicine, 42*(11), 1511–1519.

Forsterling, F. (1985). Attributional retraining: A review. *Psychological Bulletin, 98*, 495–512.

Foss, L. (2001). *The End of Modern Medicine: Biomedical Science under a Microscope.* New York: SUNY Series in Constructive Postmodern Thought.

Fournier, M., Ridder, D. de & Bensing (2002). How optimism contributes to the adaptation of chronic illness: A prospective study into the enduring effects of optimism on adaptation moderated by the controllability of chronic illness. *Personality and Individual Differences, 33*(7), 1163–1183.

Frank, A. (2002). Why study people's stories? The dialogical ethics of narrative analysis. *International Journal of Qualitative Methods, 1*(1), 109–117.

Frank, A.W. (1995). *The Wounded Storyteller.* New York: University of Chicago Press.

Frank, J.D. (1974). Psychotherapy: The restoration of morale. *American Journal of Psychiatry, 131*, 271–274.

———. (1975). The faith that heals. *Johns Hopkins Medical Journal, 137*, 127–131.

Frank, J.D. & Frank, J.B. (1991). *Persuasion and Healing.* London: The John Hopkins University Press.

Frankl, V. (1963). *Man's Search for Meaning.* New York: Washington Square Press.

French, D.P., James, D., Horne, R. & Weinman, J. (2010). Causal beliefs and behaviour change post-myocardial infarction: How are they related? *British Journal of Health Psychology, 10*(2), 167–182.

Frydenberg, E. (2004). Coping competencies: What to teach and when. *Theory and Practice, 43*(1), 14–22.

Galbraith, P.L. & Barton, B.W. (1990*). Subliminal Relaxation: Myth or Method.* Weber State University, USA. Unpublished Dissertation.

Gallacher, J.E.J., Sweetnam, P.M., Yarnell, J.W.G., Elwood, P.C. & Stansfeld, S.A. (2003). Is Type A really a trigger for coronary heart disease events? *Psychosomatic Medicine, 65*, 339–346.

Gardner, J.K., McConnell, T.R., Klinger, T.A., Herman, C.P., Hauck, C.A., et al. (2003). Quality of life and self-efficacy: Gender and diagnoses considerations for management during cardiac rehabilitation. *Journal of Cardiopulmonary Rehabilitation, 231,* 299–306.

Garro, L.C. (1994). Narrative representations of chronic illness experience: Cultural models of illness, mind and body in stories concerning the temporomandibular joint (TMJ). *Social Science and Medicine, 38,* 775–788.

Gergen, K.J. & Gergen, M.M. (1988). Narrative and the self as relationship. In L. Berkowitz (Ed.), *Advances in Experimental Social Psychology* (Vol. 21, pp. 17–56). New York: Academic Press.

Gergen, M.M. (1988). Narrative structures in social explanation. In G. Antaki (Ed.), *Analysing Everyday Explanation: A Casebook of Methods* (pp. 94–112). London: SAGE Publications.

Gerro, L.C. (1994). Narrative representations of chronic illness experience: Cultural models of illness, mind and body in stories concerning the temporomandibular joint (TMJ). *Social Science and Medicine, 38,* 775–788.

Ghadially, R. (1988). *Women in Indian Society: A Reader.* New Delhi: SAGE Publications.

Ghaeml, S.N. (2009). Editorial: The rise and fall of the biopsychosocial model. *The British Journal of Psychiatry, 195,* 3–4.

Gill, K.S. (1977). *Evolution of the Indian Economy.* New Delhi: NCERT Publication.

Gillis, C.L. (1984). Reducing family stress during and after coronary artery bypass surgery. *Nursing Clinics of the North America, 19,* 1103–1111.

Gilson, B.S., Gilson, J.S., Bergner, M., Bobbitt, R.A., Kressel, S., Pollard, W.E., et al. (1975). The sickness impact profile: Development of an outcome measure of health care. *American Journal of Public Health, 65,* 1304–1310.

Giltay, E.J., Kamphuis, M.H., Kalmijn, S., Zitman, F.G. & Kromhout, D. (2006). Dispositional optimism and the risk of cardiovascular death: The Zutphen Elderly Study. *Archieves of Internal Medicine, 166,* 431–436.

Glass, D.C. (1976). *Behaviour Patterns, Stress and Coronary Disease.* Hillsdale, NJ: Erlbaum.

Glasser, W. (1996). *Positive Addiction.* New York: Harper & Row.

Goffman, E. (1961). *Asylum: Essays on the Social Situation of Mental Patients and Other Inmates.* New York: Doubleday.

Gokhale, B.G. (1961). *Indian Thought through the Ages: A Study of Some Document Concepts.* Bombay: Asia Publishing House.

Goldiamon, I. (1975). Insider-outsider problems: A constructional approach. *Rehabilitation Psychology, 22,* 103–116.

Goldsmith, H. (1955). *A contribution of certain personality characteristics of male paraplegics to the degree of improvement in rehabilitation.* Unpublished doctoral dissertation, New York University.

Gomez, C.R., Boehmer, E.D. & Kovacs, E.J. (2005). The aging innate immune system. *Current Opinion on Immunology, 17,* 457–462.

Gore, M.S. (1968). *Urbanization and Family Change.* Bombay: Popular Prakashan.

Gore, M.S. (1985). Social support and styles of coping with stress. In S. Cohen & S.L. Syme (Eds), *Social Support and Health*. New York: Academic Press.

Grbich, C. (2004). *New Approaches in Social Research*. London: SAGE Publications.

Greenberg, L.W., Jewett, L.S., Gluck, R.S., Champion, L.A.A., Leikin, S.E., Altieri, M.F. & Liprick, R.N. (1984). Giving information for a life threatening diagnosis: Parents and oncologists perceptions. *American Journal of Diabetes Care*, *138*, 649–653.

Gupta, G.R. (1978). The joint family. In M.S. Das & P.D. Bardis (Eds), *The Family in Asia*. New Delhi: Vikas Publications.

Guthrie, E. (1996). Emotional disorder in chronic illness: psychotherapeutic interventions. *British Journal of Psychiatry*, *168*, 265–273.

Haan, N. (1977). *Coping and Defending: Processes of Self Environment Organization*. New York: Academic Press.

Hagger, M. & Orbell, S. (2003). A meta-analytic review of the common-sense model of illness representations. *Psychology and Health*, *18*, 141–184.

Hamburg, D.A. & Adams, J.E. (1967). A perspective on coping behavior: Seeking and utilizing information in major transitions. *Archives of General Psychiatry*, *17*, 277–284.

Health Information India. (1988). *Ministry of Health and Family Welfare*. New Delhi: Government of India.

Heider, F. (1958). *Psychology of Interpersonal Relations*. New York: Wiley.

Hertz, R. (1997). (Ed.). *Reflexivity and Voice*. London: SAGE Publications.

Herzlich, C. (1973). *Health and Illness: A Social Psychological Analysis*. London: Academic Press.

Hinkle, L.E. Jr. (1973). The concept of 'stress' in biological and social sciences. *Science, Medicine and Man*, *1*, 314.

Hirsch, B. (1981). Social networks and the coping process. In B. Gottlieb (Ed.), *Social Networks and Social Support*. Beverly Hills: SAGE Publications.

Hirt, E.R., McCrea, S.M. & Boris, H.I. (2003). 'I know you self-handicapped last exam': Gender differences in reactions to self-handicapping. *Journal of Personality and Social Psychology*, *84*(1), 177–193.

Holmes, T. & Rahe, R. (1967). The social readjustment rating scale. *Journal of Psychosomatic Research*, *11*, 213–218.

Holstein, J.A. & Gubrium, J.F. (2000). *The Self We Live By: Narrative Identity in Post Modern World*. New York: Oxford University Press.

House, J. & Kahn, R. (1985). Measures and concepts and social support. In S.Cohen & L. Syme (Eds), *Social Support and Health*. New York: Academic Press.

House, J., Robbins, C. & Metzner, H. (1982). The association of social relationships and activities with mortality: Perspective evidence from the Tecumseh community health study. *American Journal of Epidemiology*, *116*, 123–140.

Hunt, S.M., McEwen, J., McKenna, S.P., Backett, E.M. & Pope, C. (1984). Subjective health assessments and the perceived outcome of minor surgery. *Journal of Psychosomaic Research*, *28*(2), 105–114.

Hydén, L.C. & Antelius, E. (2011). Communicative disability and stories: Towards an embodied conception of narratives. *Health, 15,* 588–603.

Illich, I. (1974). *Medical Nemesis.* London: Calder & Boyars.

Isaac, I. & Shah, A. (2004). Sex roles and marital adjustment in Indian couples. *International Journal of Social Psychiatry, 50,* 129–141.

Jaber, F.G. & Holstein, J.A. (2009). *Analysing Narrative Reality.* Thousand Oaks, CA: SAGE Publications.

Jachuk, S.J., Brierley, H., Jachuk, S. & Willcox, P.M. (1982). The effect of hypotensive drugs on the quality of life. *Journal of the Royal College of General Practitioner, 32,* 103–105.

Jain, U.C. (1987). Attribution-behavior relationship in the context of learned helplessness. In A.K. Dalal (Ed.), *Attribution Theory and Research in India.* New Delhi: Eastern Wiley.

Janis, I.L. & Rodin, J. (1979). Attribution, control and decision-making: Social Psychology in health care. In G.C. Stone, F. Cohen & N.E. Adler (Eds), *Health Psychology.* San Francisco: Jossey-Bass.

Janoff-Bulman, R. & Wortman, C.B. (1977). Attributions of blame and coping in the 'real world': Severe accident victims react to their lot. *Journal of Personality and Social Psychology, 35,* 351–363.

Janoff-Bulman, R.J. & Lang-Gunn, L. (1986). Coping with disease and accidents: The role of self-blame attributions. In L.Y. Abramson (Ed.), *Social Cognition and Clinical Psychology: A Synthesis* (pp. 116–147). New York: Guilford Press.

Jansen, D.L., Rijken, M., Heijmans, M. & Boeschoten, E.W. (2010). Perceived autonomy and self-esteem in Dutch dialysis patients: The chronic kidney disease and renal transplantation importance of illness and treatment perceptions. *Psychology and Health, 25*(6), 733–749.

Joshi, P.C. (1988). Traditional medical system in the Central Himalayas. *The Eastern Anthropologists, 41,* 77–86.

―――. (2000). Relevance and utility of traditional medical systems (TMS) in the context of a Himalayan tribe. *Psychology and Developing Societies, 12,* 5–29.

Kakar, S. (1982). *Shaman, Mystics and Doctors: A Psychological Inquiry into India and Its Healing Traditions.* New Delhi: Oxford University Press.

―――. (1991). *The Analyst and the Mystic.* New Delhi: Viking.

―――. (2003). Psychoanalysis and Eastern spiritual traditions. *Journal of Analytic Psychology, 48,* 659–678.

Kakar, S. & Kakar, K. (2007). *The Indians: Portrait of a People.* New Delhi: Penguin.

Kanekar, S. (1988). Attribution of causal and moral responsibility: The case of a rape victim. In A.K. Dalal (Ed.), *Attribution Theory and Research.* New Delhi: Wiley Eastern Limited.

Kangas, I. (2001). Making sense of depression: Perceptions of melancholia in lay narratives. *Health Psychology, 5*(1), 76–92.

Kapoor, R.L. (2003). What is psychotherapy? Unpublished report, National Institute of Advanced Studies, Bangalore.

Kasl, S.V. & Cobb, S. (1966). Health behaviour, illness behaviour and sick role behaviour. *Arch. Environmental Health, 12,* 246–266, 531–541.

Katz, A.H. & Bender, E.I. (Eds). (1976). *The Strength in Us*. New York: Franklin Watts.

Kelley, H.H. (1967). Attribution in social psychology. *Nebraska Symposium on Motivation, 15*, 192–239.

———. (1992). Common-sense psychology and scientific psychology. *Annual Review of Psychology, 43*, 1–24.

Kessler, R.C., McLeod, J.D. & Wethington, E. (1984). The cost of caring. In I.G. Sarason & B.R. Sarason (Eds), *Social Support: Theory, Research and Applications*. The Hague: Martinus Nijhof.

Kiecolt-Glaser, J.K., Fisher, L.D., Ogrock, P., Stout, J.C., Speicher, C.E. & Glaser, R. (1987). Marital quality, marital disruption and immune function. *Psychosomatic Medicine, 9*, 13–34.

Kiev, A. (1965). The study of folk psychiatry. *International Journal of Psychology, 1*(4), 524–552.

Kirscht, J.P. (1983). Preventive health behavior: A review of research and issues. *Health Psychology, 2*, 277–301.

Kleinman, A. (1974). The cognitive structure of traditional medicinal systems. *Ethnomedicine, 27*, 27–49.

———. (1980). *Patients and Healers in the Context of Culture*. Berkeley: University of California Press.

———. (1988). *Rethinking Psychiatry: From Cultural Category to Personal Experience*. New York: Free Press.

Kleinman, A., Eisenberg, L. & Good, B. (1978). Culture, illness and care: Clinical lessons from anthro-polgic and cross-cultural research. *Annals of Internal Medicine, 88*, 251–258.

Kleinman, A. & Seeman, D. (2000). Personal experience of illness. In G.T. Albrecht, R. Fitzpatrick & S.C. Scrimshaw (Eds), *The Handbook of Social Studies in Health and Medicine* (pp. 230–242). London: SAGE Publications.

Kleinman, A. & Sung, L.H. (1979). Why do indigenous practitioners successfully heal? *Social Science and Medicine, 13*, 7–16.

Kleinman, A.K. (1974). The cognitive structure of traditional medical systems. *Ethnomedicine, 3*, 27–49.

———. (1978). Concepts and models for the comparison of medical systems. *Social Science and Medicine, 12*, 85–93.

———. (1986). *The Illness Narratives: Suffering, Healing and Human Conditions*. New York: Basic Books.

Kobasa, S.C. (1979). Stressful life events, personality, and health: An inquiry into hardiness. *Journal of Personality and Social Psychology, 37*, 1–11.

Kohli, N. (1995). *Coping with tragic life events: A study of cancer patients*. Unpublished doctoral dissertation, University of Allahabad, India.

Kokanovic, R., Butler, E., Halilovich, H., Palmer, V., Griffiths, F., Dowrick, C. & Gunn, J. (2013). Maps, models and narratives: The way people talk about depression. *Qualitative Health Research, 23*(11), 114–125.

Kornfeld, D.A. (1972). The hospital environment: Its impact on the patient. *Advances in Psychosomatic Medicine, 8*, 252–270.

Kothari, M.L. & Mehta, L. (1988). Violence in modern medicine. In A. Nandy (Ed.), *Science, Hegemony and Violence*. New Delhi: Oxford University Press.

Krantz, D.A. (1980). Cognitive processes and recovery from heart attack: A review and theoretical analysis. *Journal of Human Stress, 6*(3), 27–38.

Krishnakumar, A. (2004). An unhealthy trend. *Frontline, 21*(24), 84–85.

Kruglanski, A.W. & Orehek, E. (2007). Partitioning the domain of social influence: Dual mode and systems models and their alternatives. *Annual Review of Psychology, 58*, 291–316.

Kubler-Ross, E. (1969). *On Death and Dying*. New York: Simon & Schuster/Touch-stone.

———. (1975). *Death: The Final Stage of Growth*. Englewood Cliffs, NJ: Prentice-Hall.

Kushwah, S.S., Govil, A.K., Upadhyay, S. & Kushwah, J. (1981). A study of social stigma among leprosy patients attending leprosy clinic in Gwalior. *Leprosy in India, 53*, 84–92.

Labov, W. & Waletzky, J. (1997). Narrative analysis: Oral version of personal experience. *Journal of Narrative and Life History, 7*(1–4), (New Jersey: Lawrence Erlbaum Associates), 3–38.

Langer, E.J. (1975). The illusion of control. *Journal of Personality and Social Psychology, 32*, 311–328.

Langner, T.S. (1962). A twenty-two item screening score of psychiatric symptoms indicating impairment. *Journal of Health and Human Behaviour, 3*, 269–276.

Lazarus, R.S. (1966). *Psychological Stress and Coping Process*. New York: McGraw-Hill.

———. (1981). The stress and coping paradigm. In C. Eisdonfer, D. Cohen & A. Kleinman (Eds), *Conceptual Models of Psychopathology* (pp. 177–214). New York: Spectrum.

———. (1983). The costs and benefits of denial. In S. Bresnitz (Ed.), *Denial of Stress* (pp. 1–30). New York: International University Press.

———. (1984). On the primacy of cognition. *American Psychologist, 39*, 124–129.

———. (1993). Illusion and well-being: A social psychological perspective on mental health. *Psychological Bulletin, 103*, 56–78.

———. (2000). Toward better research on stress and coping. *American Psychologist, 55*, 665–673.

Lazarus, R.S., Averill, J.R. & Option, J. (1970). Toward a cognition. In M.B. Arnold (Ed.), *Feelings and Emotions: The Royal Symposium* (pp. 207–232). New York: Academic Press.

Leight, S.B. (2003). The application of a vulnerable population: Conceptual model of rural health. *Public Health Nursing, 20*(6), 440–448.

Lerner, M.J. (1971). Observers's evaluation of a victim: Justice, guilt, and veridical perception. *Journal of Personality and Social Psychology, 20*, 127–135.

———. (1975). Justice motive in social behaviour. *Journal of Social Issues, 31*, 1–20.

Lerner, M.J. & Mathews, G. (1967). Reactions to suffering of others under conditions of indirect responsibility. *Journal of Personality and Social Psychology*, 5, 319–325.

Leventhal, H. & Benyamini, Y. (1997). Lay beliefs about health and illness. In A. Baum, C. McManus, S. Newman, J. Weinman & R. Best (Eds), *Cambridge Handbook of Psychology, Health and Medicine*. Cambridge, UK: Cambridge University Press.

Leventhal, H., Nerenz, D.R. & Steele, D.J. (1984). Illness representations and coping with health threats. In A. Baum & J. Singer (Eds), *A Handbook of Psychology and Health* (Vol. 4, pp. 219–252). Hillsdale, NJ: Erlbaum.

Levin, J. (2009). How faith heals: A theoretical model. *Explore*, 5, 77–96.

Lieberman, M. (1982). The effects of social support on response to stress. In L. Goldberg & Breznits, S. (Eds), *Handbook of Stress*. New York: The Free Press.

Lindsey, A.M. (1993). Stress response. In V. Carrieri, A.M. Lindsey & C.M. West (Eds), *Pathophysiological Phenomena in Nursing: Human Responses to Illness* (pp. 397–419). Philadelphia, PA: W.B. Saunders.

Linkowski, D.C. (1971). A scale to measure acceptance of disability. *Rehabilitation Counseling Bulletin*, 14, 236–244.

Lipowski, Z.J. (1983). Psychosocial reactions to physical illness. *Canadian Medical Association Journal*, 128(9), 1069–1072.

Lipton, B.H. (2008). *The Biology of Belief*. New York: Hay House.

Lown, B. (2007). The commodification of health care. PNHP Newsletter (full title not available).

Lupton, D. (1994). *Medicine Is Culture: Disease and Health in Western Societies*. London: SAGE Publications.

Lusk, B. & Lash, A.A. (2005). The stress response, psychoneuroimmunology, and stress among ICU patients. *Dimensions of Critical Care Nursing*, 24(2), 25–31

Maddux, J.E. (2009). Self-efficacy: The power of believing you can. In S.J. Lopez & C.R. Snyder (Eds), *Handbook of Positive Psychology* (pp. 335–343). New York: Oxford University Press.

Major, B.N., Mueller, P. & Hildebrandt, K. (1985). Attributions, expectations, and coping with abortion. *Journal of Personality and Social Psychology*, 48, 585–599.

Malhotra, S. (2008). Psycho-oncology research in India: Current status and future directions. *Journal of the Indian Academy of Applied Psychology*, 34(1), 7–18.

Malkin, J. (2003). The business case for creating a healing environment. *Business Briefing: Hospital Engineering and Facilities Management*, 12, 1–5.

Mariott, M. (1955). *Village India: Studies in the Little Community*. Chicago: University of Chicago Press.

Markovic, M., Manderson, L. & Warren, N. (2008). Endurance and contest: Women's narratives of endometriosis. *Health*, 12(3), 349–367.

Markus, H.R. & Kitayama, S. (1991). Culture and the self: Implications for cognition, emotion and motivation. *Psychological Review*, 98, 224–253.

Mason, J.W. (1971). A re-evaluation of the concept of 'non-specificity' in stress theory. *Journal of Psychiatric Research, 8,* 323–333.

Mathews, A. & Ridgeway, V. (1981). Personality and surgical recovery: A review. *British Journal of Clinical Psychology, 20*(Pt 4), 243–260

McDowell, I. & Newwell, C. (1987). *Measuring Health: A Guide to Rating Scales and Questionnaire.* New York: Oxford University Press.

McFall, R.M. (2006). Doctoral training in clinical psychology. *Annual Review of Clinical Psychology, 2,* 21–49

McLeod, J. (1996). The emerging narrative approach to counselling and psychotherapy. *British Journal of Guidance and Counselling, 24,* 173–184.

Meichenbaum, D.H. (1977). *Cognitive-Behaviour Modification.* New York: Plenum.

Meile, R.L. (1972). The 22-item index of psychophysical disorder: Psychological or organic symptoms? *Social Science and Medicine, 6,* 125–135.

Menon, N. (2004). Refusing globalisation and the authentic nation: Feminist politics in current conjecture. *Economic and Political Weekly,* 3 January, 100–104

Meyerowitz, B.F. (1980). Psychosocial correlates of breast cancer and its treatment. *Psychological Bulletin, 87,* 108–131.

Miller, I.W. & Norman, W.H. (1979). Learned helplessness in humans: A review and attribution theory model. *Psychological Bulletin, 86,* 93–118.

Miller, W.R. & Thoresen, C.E. (2003). Spirituality, religion, and health: An emerging research field. *American Psychologist, 58,* 24–35.

Millon, T., Green, C.J. & Meagher, R.B. (1979). The MBHI: A new inventory for the psycho-diagnostician in medical settings. *Professional Psychology, 10,* 529–539.

Minuchin, S. (1974). *Families and Family Therapy.* Cambridge: Harvard University Press.

Miri, Sujata (1976). *Suffering.* Shimla, India: Indian Institute of Advanced Study.

Misra, G. (1994). Psychology of control: Cross-cultural considerations. *Journal of Indian Psychology, 12,* 8–45.

Misra, G. & Misra, S. (1986). Effect of socioeconomic background on pupil's attribution. *Indian Journal of Current Psychological Research, 1,* 77–88.

Mital, A., Desai, A. & Mital, A. (2004). Return to work after a coronary event. *Journal of Cardiopulmonary Rehabilitation, 24,* 365–373.

Molzahn, A.E. & Sheilds, L. (2008). Why is it so hard to talk about spirituality? *Canadian Nurse, 104,* 25–29.

Monroe, S.M. & Steiner, S.C. (1986). Social support and psychopathology: Interrelations with preexisting disorders, stress and personality. *Journal of Abnormal Psychology, 95,* 29–39.

Mumma, C. & McCorkle, R. (1982). Causal attributions and life threatening disease. *International Journal of Psychiatry in Medicine, 12,* 312–319.

Nanda, M. (2009). *The God Market: How Globalization Is Making India More Hindu.* New Delhi: Random House.

Neki, J.S. (1975). Psychotherapy in India: Past, present and future. *American Journal of Psychotherapy, 29,* 92–100.

News (September 1996). *APA Monitor*. Washington, D.C.: American Psychological Association.

Nicassio, P., Wallston, K., Callahan, L., Herbert, M. & Pincus, T. (1985). The measurement of helplessness in rheumatoid arthritis. The development of the arthritis helplessness index. *Journal of Rheumatology, 12*, 462–467.

Nienke, B.L. (2012). *Construction and validation of a hospital environmental rating scale*. Unpublished paper, Universiteit Twente, Germany.

O'Hara, M. (2000). Emancipatory therapeutic practices for a new era: A work of retrieval. In Kirk J. Schneider, James F.T. Bugantal & Jean Fraser Pierson (Eds), *Handbook of Humanistic Psychology*. London: SAGE Publications.

Oommen, T.K. (1991). Family research in India: Issues and priorities. In Unit for Family Studies (Ed.), *Research on Families with Problems in India*. Bombay: Tata Institute of Social Sciences Publication.

Osler, W. (1910). The faith that heals. *British Medical Journal, June 18*, 1470–1472.

Pande, N. & Naidu, R.K. (1986). Task effort and outcome orientations as moderators of stress-strain relationship. *Psychological Studies, 31*, 207–214.

———. (1992). Anasakti and health: A study of non-attachment. *Psychology and Developing Societies, 4*, 89–104.

Paranjpe, A.C. (1984). *Theoretical Psychology: The Meeting of East and West*. New York: Plenum Press.

———. (1998). *Self and Identity in Modern Psychology and Indian Thought*. New York: Plenum Press.

———. (2006). From tradition through colonialism to globalization: Reflections on the history of psychology in India. In D. Brock (Ed.), *Internationalizing the History of Psychology*. London: New York University Press.

Parham, P. (2005). *Elements of the Immune System and Their Roles in Defense: The Immune System*, 2nd ed. New York: Garland Science Publishing.

Parikh, I. & Garg, P. (1989). *The Inner Voices*. New Delhi: Concept Publishers.

Park, C.L., Chmielewski, J. & Blank, T.O. (2010). Post-traumatic growth: Finding positive meaning in cancer survivorship moderates the impact of intrusive thoughts on adjustment in younger adults. *Psycho-Oncology, 19*(11), 1139–1147.

Parson, T. (1972). Definition of illness in the light of American values and social structure. In E.G. Jaco (Ed.), *Patients, Physicians and Illness* (pp. 97–117). New York: The Free Press.

Pathak, S. (1979). *Social Welfare, Health and Family Welfare in India*. New Delhi: Marwah Publications.

Pearcy, L. (1985). Galen: A biographical sketch. Retrieved 14 September 2013, from http://course.edasu.edu/horan/ced522readings/galen/dreams/galenbio

Pedersen, S.S., Tekle, F.B., Hoogwegt, M.D., Jordaens, L. & Theuns, D.A. (2012). Shock and patient preimplantation type D personality are associated with poor health status in patients with implantable cardioverter–defibrillator. *Circ Cardiovascular Quality Outcomes, 5*, 373–380.

Pederson, S.S., Ong, A.T.L., Sonnenschein, K., Serruys, P.W., Erdman, R.A.M. & van Domburg, R.T. (2006). Type D personality and diabetes predict the onset of depressive symptoms in patients after percutaneous coronary intervention. *American Heart Journal, 151*(2), 367.e1–367.e6.

Pennebaker, J. (1991). *Opening Up: The Healing Power of Confiding in Others.* New York: Avon.

Peterson, C. (2000). Future of optimism. *American Psychologist, 55*(1), 45–55.

Peterson, C., Seligman, M.E.P. & Vaillant, G.E. (1988). Pessimistic explanatory style in a risk factor for physical illness: A thirty-five year longitudinal study. *Journal of Personality and Social Psychology, 55*, 23–27.

Petrie, K.J., Lana, A., Jago, D. & Devcich, A. (2007). Disclosures. *Current Opinion in Psychiatry, 20*(2), 163–167.

Phillips, D.P., Van Voorhees, C.A. & Ruth, T.E. (1992). The birthday: lifeline or deadline? *Psychosomatic Medicine, 54*, 532–542.

Powell, T. (1997). Consultation-liaison, psychiatry and clinical ethics. *Psychosomatics*, 38, 321–326.

Price, D.D., Finniss, D.G. & Benedetti, F. (2008). A comprehensive review of the placebo effect: Recent advances and current thought. *Annual Review of Psychology*, 59, 565–590.

Price, J. (1996). Snakes in the swamp: Ethical issues in qualitative research. In R. Josselson (Ed.), *Ethics and Process in the Narrative Study of Lives* (pp. 207–215). Thousand Oaks, CA: SAGE Publications.

Priya, Ravi K. (2010). The research relationship as a facilitator of remoralization and self-growth: Postearthquake suffering and healing. *Qualitative Health Research, 20*(4), 479–495.

Purohit, S. (2002). Faith that works. *Hindusthan Times* (20 February). Lucknow Edition.

Radhakrishnan, S. (1926, 1953). *The Hindu View of Life.* Bombay: Blakie.

Radley, A. (1994). *Making Sense of Illness.* London: SAGE Publications.

Ragland, D.R. & Brand, R.J. (1988). Type A behavior and mortality from coronary heart disease. *New England Journal of Medicine, 318*(2), 65–69.

Raina, B.L. (1990). *Health Sciences in Ancient India.* New Delhi: Commonwealth Publishers.

Ramachandran, V., Menon, S. & Arunagiri, S. (1982). Socio-cultural factors in late onset of depression. *Indian Journal of Psychiatry, 24*, 268–273.

Ramani, K.V., Mavalankar, D. & Govil, D. (Eds). (2008). *Strategic Issues and Challenges in Health Management.* New Delhi: SAGE Publications.

Rankin, J. (2002). What is narrative? Ricoeur, Bakhtin and process approaches. Concrescence: *Australian Journal of Process Thought, 3*, 1–12.

Raskin, J.D. (2002). Constructivism in psychology: Personal construct psychology, radical constructivism, and social constructionism. *American Communication Journal, 5*(3), 1–25.

Rawlett, K.E. (2011). Analytical evaluation of the health belief model and the vulnerable populations conceptual model applied to a medically underserved, rural population. *International Journal of Applied Science and Technology, 1*(2), 15–21.

Reid, D. (1984). Participating control and the chronic illness adjustment process. In H. Lefcourt (Ed.), *Research with the Locus of Control Construct: Extensions and Limitations* (pp. 361–369). New York: Academic Press.

Rennie, D.L., Phillips, J.R. & Quartaro, G.K. (1988). Grounded theory: A promising approach to conceptualization in psychology? *Canadian Psychology*, 29(2), 139–150.

Reuben, B.F. & Omorilewa, A.F. (1991). Perception of situational stress associated with hospitalization among selected Nigerian patients. *Journal of Advanced Nursing*, 16(4), 469–474.

Ricoeur, P. (1991). Life in quest of narrative. In D. Wood (Ed.), *On Paul Ricoeur: Narrative and Interpretation*. London: Routledge.

Riessman, C.K. (2008). *Narrative Methods for the Human Sciences*. Los Angeles, CA: SAGE Publications.

Roberts, N., Smith, R., Bennett, S., Cape, J., Norton, R. & Kilburn, P. (1984). Health beliefs and rehabilitation after lumbar disc surgery. *Journal of Psychosomatic Research*, 28, 139–144.

Rosenbaum, M. (1983). Learned resourcefulness as a behavioral repertoire for the self-regulation of internal events: Issues and speculations. In M. Rosenbaum, L.M. Franks & Y. Jaffe (Eds), *Perspectives on Behavior Therapy in the Eighties*. New York: Springer.

———. (Ed.). (1990). *Learned Resourcefulness: On Coping Skills, Self-control, and Adaptive Behavior*. New York: Springer

Rosenbaum, M. & Ben-Ari, K. (1985). Learned helplessness and learned resourcefulness: Effects of noncontingent success and failure on Individuals in self-control skills. *Journal of Personality and Social Psychology*, 48, 198–215.

Rosenman, R.H., Friedman, M., Straus, R., Jenkins, C.D., Zyzanski, S.J. & Wurm, M. (1970). Coronary heart disease in the Western Collaborative Group Study. A follow-up experience of 4 and one-half years. *Journal of Chronic Diseases*, 23(3), 173–190.

Rosenstock, I.M. (1966). Why people use health services. *Milbank Memorial Fund Quaterly*, 44, 94–124.

———. (1974). The health belief model and preventive health behaviour. *Health Education Monographs*, 2, 354–386.

Rothbaum, F., Morling, B. & Rusk, N. (2009). How goals and beliefs lead people into and out of depression. *Review of General Psychology*, 13, 302–314.

Rothbaum, F., Weiss, J.R. & Snyder, S.S. (1982). Changing the world and changing the self: A two process model of perceived control. *Journal of Personality and Social Psychology*, 42, 5–37.

Rotter, J.B. (1966). Generalized expectancies for internal versus external control of reinforcement. *Psychological Monographs*, 80, 1–28.

Roussi, P. & Advi, E. (2008). Meaning making and chronic illness: Cognitive and narrative approaches. *Hellenic Journal of Psychology*, 5, 147–178.

Rubin, D.C. (Ed.). (1986). *Autobiographical Memory*. Cambridge, England: Cambridge University Press.

Sahin, B., Yilmaz, F. & Lee, K.H. (2007). Factors affecting inpatient satisfaction: Structural equation modeling. *Journal of Medical System, 31*(1), 9–16.

Scheier, M.F. & Carver, C.S. (1985). Optimism, coping and health: Assessment and implications of generalized outcome expectancies. *Health Psychology, 4,* 219–247.

Scheier, M.F., Weintraub, J.K. & Carver, C.S. (1986). Divergent strategies of optimists and pessimists. *Journal of Personality and Social Psychology, 51,* 1257–1264.

Schleifer, S.J., Eckholdt, H.M., Cohen, J. & Keller, S.E. (1993). Analysis of partial variance (APV) as a statistical approach to control day to day variation in immune assays. *Brain Behaviour Immunology, 7,* 243–252.

Schleifer, S.J., Keller, S.E., Bond, R.N., Cohen, J. & Stein, M. (1989). Major depressive disorder and immunity: Role of age, sex, severity and hospitalization. *Archives of General Psychiatry, 46,* 81–87.

Schussler, G. (1992). Coping strategies and individual meaning of illness. *Social Science and Medicine, 34,* 427–432.

Schwartz, B. (2000). Self-determination: The tyranny of freedom. *American Psychologist, 55*(1), 79–88.

Segerstrom, S.C. & Miller, G.E. (2004). Psychological stress and the human immune system: Meta-analytic study of 30 years of inquiry. *Psychological Bulletin, 130*(4), 1–37, 601–630.

Seligman, M.E.P. (1975). *Helplessness: On Depression, Development and Death.* San Francis: Faceman.

Sensky, T. (1997). Causal attribution in physical illness. *Journal of Psychosomatic Research, 43*(6), 565–573.

Selye, K. (1976). *The Stress of Life,* 2nd ed. New York: Mcgraw-Hill.

Sethi, B.B. & Sharma, M. (1982). Family factors in psychiatric illness. In A. Kiev & A.V. Rao (Eds), *Readings in Transcultural Psychiatry.* Madras: Higginbotham.

Seymour, S.C. (1999). *Women, Family, and Child Care in India: A World in Transition.* Cambridge: Cambridge University Press.

Shah, M. (2010). *Waiting for Health Care: A Survey of a Public Hospital in Kolkata.* New Delhi: ICMR.

Sharma, M. & Srivastava, A. (1991). The family, social network and mental health. In Unit for Family Studies (Ed.), *Research on Families with Problems in India.* Bombay: Tata Institute of Social Sciences Publication.

Sharma, S. & Misra, G. (2012). Health psychology: Progress and challenges. In G. Misra (Ed.), *Psychology in India: Clinical and Health Psychology* (Vol. 3). New Delhi: Pearson.

Shaver, K.G. (1970). Defensive attribution: Effects of severity and relevance on the responsibility assigned for an accident. *Journal of Personality and Social Psychology, 14,* 101–113.

Sheikh, A.A., Kunzendorf, R.G. & Sheikh, K.S. (1989). Healing images: From ancient wisdom to modern science. In A.A. Sheikh & K.S. Sheikh (Eds), *Healing East and West* (pp. 470–515). New York: John Wiley & Sons.

Shontz, F.C. (1975). *The Psychological Aspects of Physical Illness and Disability.* New York: McMillan.

Shorer, E. (2005). The history of the biopsychosocial approach in medicine: Before and after Angel. In P. White (Ed.), *Biopsychosocial Medicine: An Integrated Approach to Understand Illness* (pp. 1–19). Oxford, UK: Oxford University Press.

Shorter, E. (2005). The history of the biopsychosocial approach in medicine: before and after Engel. In P. White (Ed.), *Biopsychosocial Medicine. An Integrated Approach to Understanding Illness* (pp. 1–21). New York: Oxford University Press.

Shumaker, S.A. & Reizenstein, J.E. (1981). Environmental factors affecting inpatient stress in acute care. In G.W. Evans (Ed.), *Environment Stress* (pp. 179–223). London: Cambridge University Press.

Siegel, B.S. (1986). *Love, Medicine and Miracles.* London: Arrow Books.

———. (1991). *Peace, Love and Healing.* London: Arrow Books.

Silver, R.L. & Wortman, C.B. (1980). Coping with undesirable life event. In J. Garber & M.E.P. Seligman (Eds), *Human Helplessness: Theory and Applications.* New York: Academic Press.

Sinding, C. & Wiernikowski, J. (2008). Disruption foreclosed: Older women's cancer narratives. *Health: An Interdisciplinary Journal for the Social Study of Health, Illness and Medicine, 12*(3), 389–411.

Singh, A. (1998). *Psycho-social study of surgical patients.* Unpublished doctoral dissertation, University of Allahabad, India.

Singh, A.K. (1987). *Role of causal and cosmic beliefs in the psychological recovery of tuberculosis patients.* Unpublished Master's dissertation, University of Allahabad, Allahabad, India.

Singh, M. & Singh, G. (1999). A Study on family and psychosocial health status of middle-aged working women of Varanasi city. *Indian Journal of Clinical Psychology, 26*(2), 246–249.

Sinha, D. (1982). *Some recent changes in the Indian families and their implications for socialization.* Paper presented at the conference on 'Changing Family in the Changing World' organized by the German Commission for UNESCO, Munich.

———. (1988). The family scenario in a developing country and its implications for mental health. In P. Dasen, J.W. Berry & N. Sartorious (Eds), *Health and Cross-cultural Psychology.* Beverly Hills: SAGE Publications.

Singh, R. (2011). *Psychological Models of Illness.* New Castle, US: Cambridge Scholars Publishing.

Sinha, Y., Jain, U.C. & Pandey, J. (1980). Attribution of causality of poverty. *Journal of Social and Economic Studies, 3,* 349–359.

Sixth Five Year Plan. (1986). *The Sixth Five Year Plan.* New Delhi: Government of India Publication.

Slater, J. & Depue, R.A. (1980). The contributions of environmental events and social support to serious suicide attempts in primary depressive disorder. *Journal of Abnormal Psychology, 90,* 275–285.

Smith, B. & Sparkes, A.C. (2011). Exploring multiple responses to a chaos narrative. *Health*, 15, 38–53.

Smith, J. & Crawford, L. (2004). Report of findings from the practice and professional issues survey Spring 2003. *National Council of State Boards of Nursing*, 4(15): http://www.ncsbn.org/pdfs/RB15_SO3PPI_ESforWeb.pdf

Smith, T.R. (2004). Narrative and consciousness. *Journal of Consciousness Studies*, 11(5), 146–155.

Smith, T.W. & Ruiz, J.M. (2002). Psychosocial influences on the development and course of coronary heart disease: Current status and implications for research and practice. *Journal of Consulting and Clinical Psychology*, 70, 548–568.

Sodani, P.R. & Sharma, K. (2011). Investigative services at public hospital to improve quality of services. *National Journal of Community Medicine*, 2(3), 405.

Solomon, G.F. (1969). Emotions, stress and Central Nervous System, and immunity. *Annals of New York Academy of Sciences*, 168, 335–343.

Sonney, J.L. & Janoff, D.S. (1982). Attributions and the maintenances of behavior change. In C. Antaki & C.R. Brewin (Eds), *Attributions and Psychological Change*. London: Academic Press.

Speedling, E.J. (1982). *Heart Attack: The Family Response at Home and in the Hospital*. New York: Tavistock.

St. Lous, P., Carter, W.B. & Eisenberg, M.S. (1982). Prescribing CPR: A survey of physicians. *American Journal of Public Health*, 72, 1158–1160.

Stanton, A.L., Collins, C.A. & Sworowski, L.A. (2001). Adjustment to chronic illness: Theory and research. In A. Baum & T.A. Revenson (Eds), *Handbook of Health Psychology* (pp. 387–403). Mahwah, NJ: Erlbaum.

Stefen, E. (2005). Pharmaceutical citizenship: Antidepressant marketing and the promise of demarginalization in India. *Anthropology & Medicine*, 12(3), 239–254.

Sternbach, R.A. (1978). *Pain: A Psycho Physiological Analysis*. New York: Academic Press.

Stevens, P.E. & Doerr, B. (1997). Trauma of discovery: women's narratives of being informed they are HIV-infected. *AIDS Care*, 9, 523–538.

Stichler, J. (2001). Creating healing environments in critical care units. *Critical Care Nursing Quarterly*, 24(3), 1–20.

Stone, A.A., Bovbjerg, D.H., Neale, J.M., Napoli, A. & Valdimarsdottir, H. (1992). Development of common cold symptoms following experimental rhinovirus infection is related to prior stressful life events. *Behavioural Medicine*, 8, 115–120.

Stone, A.A., Cox, D.S., Valdimarsdottir, H., Jandorf, L. & Neale, J.M. (1987). Evidence that secretory IgA antibody is associated with daily mood. *Journal of Personality and Social Psychology*, 52, 988–993.

Storey, A.H., Jr. (2008). *The impact of biculturalism on human learned helplessness with Northern Plains Native Americans*. Unpublished PhD dissertation, University of North Dakota, USA.

Stuhlmiller, C.M. (2001). Narrative methods in qualitative research: Potential for therapeutic transformation. In K.R. Gilbert (Ed.), *The Emotional Nature of Qualitative Research* (pp. 63–80). Boca Raton, Florida: CRC Press.

Schussler, G. (1992). Coping strategies and individual meanings of illness. *Social Science and Medicine, 34*, 427–432.

Sweeney, P.D., Anderson, K. & Bailey B. (1986). Attributional style in depression a meta-analytic review. *Journal of Personality and Social Psychology, 50*(5), 974–991.

Tagliacozzo, L., Lashof, D.B. & Ima, K. (1984). Nurso intervention and patient behavior: An experimental study. *American Journal of Public Health, 64*, 596–603.

Talbott, E., Kuller, L.H., Perper, J. & Murphy, P.A. (1981). Sudden unexpected death in women. *American Journal of Epidemiology, 114*, 671–682.

Tanner-Smith, E. (2010). Evaluating the health belief model: A critical review of studies predicting mammograpohic and pap screening. *Social theory and Health, 8*(1), 95–125.

Taylor, S. (1983). Adjustment to threatening events: A theory of cognitive adaptation. *American Psychologist, 41*, 1161–1173.

———. (2006). *Health Psychology.* New York: McGraw-Hill.

Taylor, S.E. (1979). Hospital patient behaviour: Reactance, helplessness, or control? *Journal of Social Issues, 35*, 156–184.

———. (1984). The developing field of health psychology. In A. Baum, S.E. Taylor & J.E. Singer (Eds), *Handbook of Psychology and Health, Vol. 4: Social Psychological Aspects of Health* (pp. 1–22). Hillsdale, NJ: Erlbaum.

Taylor, S.E. & Brown, J.D. (1994). Illusion and well-being: A social psychological perspective on mental health. *Psychological Bulletin, 103*(2), 193–210.

Taylor, S.E., Crocker, J., Fiske, S.T., Sprinzen, M. & Winkler, J. (1979). The generalizability of salience effects. *Journal of Personality and Social Psychology, 37*, 357–368.

Taylor, S.E., Lichtman, R.R. & Wood, J.V. (1984). Attributions, beliefs about control, and adjustment to breast cancer. *Journal of Personality and Social Psychology, 46*, 489–502.

Thompson, S.C. (1981). Will it hurt less if I can control it? A complex answer to a simple question. *Psychological Bulletin, 90*, 89–101.

Tilvis, R.S., Laitala, V., Routasalo, P., Strandberg, T.E. & Pitkala, K.H. (2012). Positive life orientation predicts good survival prognosis in old age. *Archieves of Gerontology, 55*(1), 133–137.

Ulmer, A., Range, L.M. & Smith, P.C. (1989). *Purpose in life: A moderator of recovery from bereavement.* Paper presented at the 97th Annual Convention of the American Psychological Association, New Orleans. LA.

VandenBos, G.R. (Ed.). (1996). Outcome assessment of psychotherapy. *American Psychologist, 51* (10), 1005–1006.

Varma, V. (1989). *A psychosocial study of the spouses of cancer patients.* Unpublished Master's dissertation, University of Allahabad.

Vaughn, L.M., Jacquez, F. & Baker, R.C. (2009). Cultural health attributions, beliefs, and practices: Effects on healthcare and medical education. *Open Medical Education Journal, 2,* 64–74.

VHAI. (1991). *India's Health Status.* New Delhi: Voluntary Health Association of India.

Vishwanathasn, S. (April 3, 1998). A celebrations of difference: Science and democracy in India. *Science, 280,* 42–43.

Walker, J. (2006). The problem with beliefs. www.nobeliefs.com/beliefs.htm

Walsters, E. (1966). Assignment of responsibility for an accident. *Journal of Personality and Social Psychology, 3,* 73–79.

Wampold, B.E. (2001). *The Great Psychotherapy Debate: Models, Methods and Funding.* Mahwah: NJ, Erlbaum.

Watts, A. (1975). *Psychotherapy East and West.* New York: Vintage Books.

Weary, G., Stanley, M.A. & Harvey, J.H. (1989). *Attribution.* New York: Springer-Verlag.

Weber, M. (1958). From Max Weber. In H. Gerth & C.W. Mills (Eds), *The Religion of India: The Sociology of Hinduism and Buddhism.* New York: Oxford University Press.

Weiner, B. (1985). 'Spontaneous' causal thinking. *Psychological Bulletin, 97,* 74–84.

Weiner, B., Russell, D. & Lerman, D. (1978). Affective consequences of causal ascriptions. In J.H. Harvey, W.J. Ickes & R.F. Kidd (Eds), *New Directions in Attribution Research* (Vol. 2). Hillsdale, NJ: Erlbaum.

Weisman, A.D. & Worden, J.E. (1975). Psychosocial analysis of cancer deaths. *Omega, 6,* 61–75.

Weiss, G.L. & Lonnquist, L.E. (1996). *The Sociology of Health, Healing and Illness.* New Jersey: Prentice-Hall.

Weiss, L.G. (2008). Toward the mastery of resiliency. *Canadian Journal of School Psychology, 23,* 127–137.

Weiss, M.G., Sharma, S.D., Gaur, R.K., Sharma, J.S., Desai, A. & Doongaji, D.R. (1986). Traditional concepts of mental disorder among Indian psychiatric patients: Preliminary report of work in progress. *Social Science and Medicine, 23*(4), 379–386.

Weller, D.J. & Miller, P.M. (1976). Emotional reactions of patient's family, and staff in acute care period of spinal cord injury: Part 1. *Social Work in Health Care, 2,* 369–377.

Westbrook, M.T. & Viney, L.L. (1982). Patterns of anxiety in the chronically ill. *British Journal of Medical Psychology, 55*(1), 87–95.

White, M. (2007). *Maps of Narrative Practice.* New York: W.W. Norton & Co.

White, R.W. (1959). Motivation reconsidered: The concept of competence. *Psychological Review, 66,* 297–333.

WHO. (2003). *Adherence to Long-term Therapies: Evidence for Action.* Geneva: World Health Organisation.

———. (2010). *Healthy Hospitals, Healthy Planet, Healthy People: Addressing Climate Change in health Care Setting.* Geneva: World Health Organization.

Williams, G. (2000). Knowledge narratives. *Anthropology and Medicine, 7*, 135–144.

Williams, R., Zyzanski, S.J. & Wright, A.L. (1992). Life events and daily hassles and uplifts as predictors of hospitalization and outpatient visitation. *Social Science & Medicine, 34*(7), 763–768.

Willis, L., Thomas, P., Garry, P.J. & Goodwin, J. (1987). A prospective study of response to stressful life events in initially healthy elders. *Journal of Gerontology, 42*, 627–630.

Winer, B.J. (1971). *Statistical Principles in Experimental Design.* Tokyo: McGraw-Hill Kogakusha Ltd.

Wondrock, W. & Taylor, S. (2008). Male caregiving of a spouse with Alzheimer's disease: A narrative of care. *Practice Reflexions, 3*(1), 29–39.

Wong, P.T.P. & Weiner, B. (1981). When people ask 'why' questions and the heuristics of attributional research. *Journal of Personality and Social Psychology, 40*, 650–663.

Wortman, C.B. (1983). *Social support and the cancer patient.* Paper presented at the annual meeting of the American Cancer Society, St. Petersburg Beach, FL.

Wortman, C.B. & Brehm, J.W. (1975). Responses to uncontrollable outcomes: An integration of reactance theory and the learned helplessness model. In L. Berkowitz (Ed.), *Advances in Experimental Social Psychology* (Vol. 8). New York: Academic Press.

Wortman, C.B. & Lehman, D.R. (1985). Reactions to victims of life crises: Support attempts that fail. In I.G. Sarason & B.R. Sarason (Eds), *Social Support: Theory, Research and Application.* Dordrecht, The Netherlands: Martinus Nijhoff.

Wujastyk, D. (1998). *The Roots of Ayurveda.* New Delhi: Penguin Books.

Young, M., Benjamin, B. & Wallis, C. (1963). Mortality of the widowers. *Lancet, 2*, 454.

Zukier, H. & Pepitone, A. (1984). Social males and strategies in prediction: Some determinants of the use of base rate information. *Journal of Personality and Social Psychology, 50*, 1–14.

Index

Acceptance of Disability (AD) Scale, 112
accident victims, psychological recovery
    of, study on role of beliefs in, 73–76
    causal beliefs, 79–81
    data collection, 77–78
    indices of psychological recovery,
        81–85
    psychological stress experienced,
        78–79
    questionnaire, 77
    sample, 76–77
adaptive immune system, 11
adjustment, in chronic disease, 110–112
affective reactions, 42–43
affective responses, repatterning of, 209
anniversary effect, 34
antibiotics, development of, 3, 6
antigens, 10
anxiety, chronic illness and, 43
APA Monitor, 212–213
attributional beliefs, 52
attributional model of psychological
    recovery, 52, 66–69
    causal and recovery attributions in,
        67–69
    human nature in, assumptions
        about, 66–67
    psychological recovery, factors in, 69
    theoretical approaches and (see
        cognitive approaches)
attribution therapy, 52
attribution to Karma, 64. See also
    principle of Karma

autobiographical memory, 160
Ayurvedic science, 23, 35

Bandura's self-efficacy theory, 59–60
behavioural control, 39–40
belief in a just world, 99–100
belief in God, 101
belief in Karma, influence of, 100–101
Biology of Beliefs, 208
biomedical model, of health care, 5, 6–7
    disease and body in, 6
    drug therapy in, role of, 6
    patient in, 6
    preventive health care and, 6
bio-medicine, development in area of, 3
Brehm's theory of reactance, 54–55
buffering effects, 190

cancer-prone personality, 17
Cartesian principle, 20
causal attributions, 63–65
causal beliefs, 86
causal search, 62–66
central themes, 165
chronic disease, 26–27
    acceptance of diagnosis of, 28, 37
    and affective reactions, 42–43
    causes of deaths due to, 26
    and chronic illness, 27
    compliance with treatment regimen,
        43–46
    definition of, 26
    depression in, 28–29

diagnosis and immediate reaction, 36–37
  families, affect on, 47
  initial reaction to, 28
  living with, 46–49
  meaning to illness, 37–39
  onset of illness, 36
  personal control and, 39–42
  prevalence of, 26
  psychological response to, 27–28
  research on people and, 29–30
  self-management of, 46
chronic disease, psychological adjustment to, study on, 87–90
  beliefs and psychological adjustment, 94–95
  causal beliefs about disease, 92–93
  discussion, 95–98
  method used, 90–92
  procedure, 91–92
  questionnaire, 91
  recovery beliefs, 93
  results, 92–95
  sample, 90
chronic illness, 27. *See also* chronic disease
clinical psychology, 5
cognitive adaptation theory, 56
cognitive approaches, 52, 53
  Bandura's self-efficacy theory, 59–60
  Brehm's theory of reactance, 54–55
  common sense model of illness perception, 58–59
  Hindu doctrine of Karma, 60–62
  Lazarus theory of cognitive appraisal, 53–54
  Taylor's theory of cognitive adaptation, 56
  theories of learned helplessness and learned optimism, 56–57
  theory of learned resourcefulness and resilience, 57–58
  Weiner's attributional theory of motivation and emotions, 55–56

cognitive control, 40
cognitive orientation, 15–16
common sense model, of illness perception, 58–59
community healing, 209
community health programmes, failure of, reasons for, 24
compensatory model, 66
compliance with treatment regimen, in chronic illness, 43–46
control beliefs, 39
  behavioural control, 39–40
  cognitive control, 40
  decision control, 40
  information control, 40
  retrospective control, 40
control over self, 89
control related beliefs, 89
coping strategies, 54
core themes, 165
cosmic beliefs, 87–88. *See also* chronic disease, psychological adjustment to, study on
cultural beliefs, xi
  chronic disease, role in, 50 (*see also* chronic disease)
  and health behaviour, 3–4
  and recovery beliefs, 65

decision control, 40
depression
  in chronically ill, 28–29, 43
  effect of, 12
  pessimistic explanatory style and, 15
Descartian logic of mind–body dualism, 4
descriptive themes, 165
disease
  and illness, distinction between, 21
  and suffering, Indian perspective on, 34–36
disease-related attributions, 52
doctor–patient communication, 133–134

Ellich, Ivan, 3
emotions, repatterning of, 209
enlightenment model, 66
ethical considerations, in narrative
   research, 165–168
   free and informed consent, 166
   narrative ownership, 167
   privacy and anonymity, 166–167
expectation-related affective reactions, 55

families, vulnerable, 193–195
family, role of, in chronic illness,
   185–186
   family support and successful
      coping, 188–190
   implications for family intervention,
      195–196
   as primary care giver, 186–188
   support, failure of, 190–193
folk healers, 31, 198. *See also* folk
   healing
folk healing, 197–200
   healers as medium, 202–203
   holistic orientation, 200–201
   and public health programmes,
      212–214
   sacred therapies, 201–202
   socio-centric treatment, 203–204
folk therapies, scientific basis of,
   204–206
   broadening domain of experience,
      208–209
   building positive social ethos,
      211–212
   creating healthy imageries, 209–210
   faith healing, 206–207
   repatterning of affective responses,
      209
   subliminal healing messages, 207–208
free-floating interviews, 159–160

general adaptation syndrome, 13
God's will, 21, 63, 65–66, 81, 83, 88,
   95–97

guru–*chela* relationship, therapeutic
   value of, 203

hardiness, 18
healing
   definition of, 197
   traditional, 198–200, 205 (*see also*
      folk healing)
healing environment, role of, in
   recovery, 130
healing institutions, 4
health
   concept of, 3, 4, 20
   cultural beliefs on, effect of, 3–4
   WHO's definition of, 23
health belief model, by Rosenstock, 21,
   44–45
health beliefs
   and affective reactions, 42–43
   functional nature of, 33–34
   of Indian people, 32–33
   meaning of, 31–33
   of patients, need of study of, 29–30
health care, 4
health-care systems, sectors of, 30
   folk sector, 31
   popular sector, 30
   professional sector, 31
health psychologists, role of, 5
health psychology, 5
   growth of, 5
Health Psychology, 5
healthy and chronically sick women,
   narrative study of, 169–173, 184
   gender-specific imageries, 178–179
   location of identity, 176–177
   narrative sessions, 174–176
   participants, 173–174
   results and discussion, 176–184
   sharing and self-disclosure,
      183–184
   themes of uprooting, 179–180
   tradition *vs.* modernity, 182–183
   world of relationships, 180–182

healthy illusions, 34
heart disease, Type A behaviour and,
    5, 16, 17
helplessness, chronic illness and, 43
Hindu doctrine of Karma, 60–62
hospitalization. *See also* perceived
    hospital environment and patients'
    emotive reactions, linkages between,
    study on
    fear from, 129
    infections acquired during, 130–131
    long-term, effects of, 130
    patients' coping reactions to,
        134–136
    stresses related to, 129–130
hospital model, 66
hospitals, in India, 131–132
    condition of, studies on, 132
    depersonalized treatment at,
        132–133
    doctor-patient communication in,
        133–134

identity construction, in process of
    narration, 156
illness, meaning of, 37–39
illness narratives, 155–159
    analysis of, 162–165
illness perceptions, 38
illusion of control, 41
imageries, healthy, creation of,
    209–210
immune system
    adaptive, 11
    function of, 10–11
    stress on, effect of, 11–12
45-item Implicit Models of Illness
    Questionnaire (IMIQ), 38
Indian Council of Medical Research,
    132
Indonesian health services, 24
information control, 40

just world hypothesis, 75, 99–100

Kobasa, Suzanne, 18

Langner's 22-item scale, 110
Lazarus theory of cognitive appraisal,
    53–54
learned helplessness, theory of, 56–57
learned optimism, 57
learned resourcefulness, 48, 74
learned resourcefulness, theory of,
    57–58
life events, stressful, 13–15
lymphocytes, 10–11

meditation, 206
mental and physical health, 4
mental health and family support,
    relationship between, 188–189
Millon Behavioral Health Inventory
    (MBHI), 112
mind and body, relationship between, 4
moral model, 66
mortality rate, stress and, 13
myocardial infarction (MI), beliefs
    about world and recovery from,
    study on, 99–102
    discussion, 106–108
    interview schedule, 102–103
    method used, 102–103
    procedure, 103
    results, 104–106
    sample, 102

'naïve psychologists', 159
narrative researcher, 161–162
narratives, in health research,
    153–154. *See also* illness narratives;
    storytelling
    big stories and small stories, 154
    and ethical considerations, 165–168
    popularity of, reason for, 155
    researcher, role of, 161–162

optimistic beliefs, 16
Osler, William, 206

pain, in chronic illnesses, 46–47
perceived hospital environment and
    patients' emotive reactions, linkages
    between, study on, 135
    data collection, 138
    discussion, 143–145
    interview schedule, 137–138
    measure of coping with hospital
        stresses, 140–143, 148–149
    method used, 136–138
    objectives of, 135–136
    operationalization of two measures,
        136–137
    perceived hospital environment
        scale, 138–140, 146–147
    results, 138–143
    sample of hospital patients, 136
personal control, belief in, 39–42. *See
    also* control beliefs
personality dispositions, and health,
    16–18
    hardiness, 18
    sense of coherence, 18
    Type A personality, 16, 17
    Type B personality, 16–17
    Type C personality, 17
    Type D personality, 17–18
physical rehabilitation, of chronically ill
    patients, 47–48
'a pill for every ill', 6
placebo effects, 9–10
positive life orientation, 16
'The Powerful Placebo' (paper), 8
primary appraisal, 53
primary care giver, family as,
    186–188
primary control, 40
primary health care, 212
primary health centres (PHCs), 212
principle of Karma, 74, 75, 84, 88,
    96–97, 100
progressive narrative, 157
psychological factors, and physical
    diseases, 5

psychological recovery, 50–51, 75,
    109
    of accident victims with physical
        disability (*see* accident victims,
        psychological recovery of, study
        on role of beliefs in)
    attributes of, 111
    attributional model of, 51–52
        (*see also* attributional model of
        psychological recovery)
    development of measure of,
        113–114 (*see also* psychological
        recovery scale, development of,
        study on)
    measures of, scales for, 110, 112
    and physical recovery, 109–110
psychological recovery scale,
    development of, study on, 113–114
    background variables and
        psychological recovery, 120–121
    data collection, 117
    discussion, 121–123
    item analysis, 117–119
    measure of psychological recovery,
        development of, 114–116,
        124–127
    method used, 114–116
    results, 117–121
    sample, 116–117
    shorter versions of scale, 119, 128
psychological stress
    brain chemicals, effect on, 12
    and diseases, 5, 8, 12–13
    and immune functioning, 10–12
    three-phase reaction to, 8
psychomedical approach, to patient
    care, 19–24. *See also* psychomedical
    model of health care
psychomedical model of health care,
    19–20
    curing and healing, distinction
        between, 22–23
    mind and body in, unity of, 20
    patient in, 20, 21

patient–practitioner relationship in, 22
people's reaction to sickness and recovery, 21–22
practical implications of, 24
socio-cultural beliefs, impact of, 20–21
Psychosocial Adjustment to Illness Scale (PAIS), 112
psychosocial rehabilitation, of chronically ill patients, 48
psychosomatic illness, 8–10
psychosomatogenic families, 194
public health, 24
public health programmes, folk healing in, 212–214

reactance, 54
Brehm's theory of, 54–55
reappraisal, 53
recovery beliefs, 65–66, 86–87
reflexivity, 161–162
regressive narrative, 157
resilience, 58
retrospective control, 40
Rotter's theory of locus of control, 89
Russian Formalist School, 162

sacredness of healing practices, 201–202
Sankhya Karika, 35
The Schedule of Recent Experiences, 14
secondary appraisal, 37, 53
secondary control, 40
self-blame, 88, 97, 98, 100
self-efficacy, 59
collective, 60
perceived, 59–60
theory of, 59–60
self-esteem-related affective reactions, 55
self-help group, 49
self-help programmes, 49

self-management, of chronic illness, 46
sense of coherence (SOC), 18, 156
Shamans, Mystics and Doctors, 198
Sickness Impact Profile (SIP), 112
social support, 188–190
socio-cultural aspects of medicine, 4
somatoform illnesses, 9
stability narrative, 157
storytelling, 155
motives behind, 157–158
sessions, 159–160
stress
and body's immune system, 10–12
defined, 13
and disease, 14
negative life events and, 13–15
Selye's biological model of, 13–14
stress inoculation programme, 48–49
stressors
acute, 11–12
chronic, 12
daily hassles, 15
naturalistic, 12
suffering
and disease, Sankhya viewpoint on, 35–36
Indian perspective on, 34–35

Taylor's theory of cognitive adaptation, 56
thematic analysis, 164–165
theory of Karma, 135
therapeutic storytelling, 155
tragic events, psychological recovery in, 73–74. See also accident victims, psychological recovery of, study on role of beliefs in
Type A personality, 5, 16, 17
Type B behaviour pattern, 16–17
Type C personality, 17
Type D personality, 17–18

vulnerable families, 193–195

Weiner's attributional theory of
motivation and emotions, 55–56
women in India, 169
changes in life of, 170
life events of, narratives of, 173 (*see also* healthy and chronically sick women, narrative study of)

in mid-life crises, 170–172
roles played by, 169
social construal of self, 172
'work of worrying', 135
world beliefs, 101, 106–108

yoga, 35, 206

About the Author

Ajit K Dalal is Professor of Psychology at the University of Allahabad, India. He had obtained his Master's degrees in Mathematics (1971) and Psychology (1974). He earned his Doctor of Philosophy degree (1978) from Indian Institute of Technology, Kanpur.

Professor Dalal had received the Fulbright Senior Fellow in 1982 and worked at the University of California, Los Angeles, and at the University of Michigan, Ann Arbor. He was also a recipient of the UGC Career Award (1990–1993), Rockefeller Foundation Award (1992) and ICSSR Senior Research Fellowship (1998 and 2012). He was an adjunct Professor at Queen's University, Canada (1992–1998) and was visiting faculty at several institutions, including National Institute of Health and Family Welfare, New Delhi, Indian Institute of Management, Ahmedabad, and Calcutta University, Kolkata. He was the editor of an international journal *Psychology and Developing Societies* (2001–2011), and is on the editorial board of several journals.

Professor Dalal has published his work in the areas such as causal attribution, health beliefs and healing traditions of India and Indian psychology. He has published about 90 research articles and book chapters. He published several books, prominent among them are: *Attribution Theory and Research* (1988), *New Directions in Indian Psychology* (vol. 1) (with G. Misra, 2002), *Social Dimensions of Health* (with S. Ray, 2005), *Handbook of Indian Psychology* (with K.R. Rao and A.C. Paranjpe, 2008), *New Directions in Health Psychology* (with R. Misra, 2011), and *Qualitative Research on Well-Being and Self-Growth: Contemporary Indian Perspectives* (with R. Priya, 2013).